MEDICINE IN THE UNITED STATES
AND THE SOVIET UNION

Medicine in the United States and the Soviet Union

A Comparative and Critical Study

By

DR. GEORGE A. TABAKOV

Formerly:

Chief of the Pediatric Division, County Hospital, Sofia, Bulgaria.

Chief of the Pediatric Division, National Bank Employees Hospital, Sofia, Bulgaria.

Founder and Physician-in-Chief of the Bulgarian Hospital in Salonika, Greece, under the auspices of the International Red Cross (during World War II).

Physician-in-Chief of the Infectious Hospital, Sofia, Bulgaria.

Editor of *Pediatrics*, Sofia.

Editor-in-Chief of *Contemporary Medicine*, Sofia.

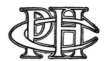

THE CHRISTOPHER PUBLISHING HOUSE

BOSTON, U.S.A.

PRINTED IN
THE UNITED STATES OF AMERICA

FOREWORD

Ever since the first Sputnik, I was impressed that the Americans are developing a sense of inferiority. It must be because they do not realize the truth about themselves and their enemy. They are being influenced by an exaggerated propaganda concerning the degree of culture, science, progress and possibilities of the USSR. The assaults throughout the globe against Americanism, Americans and their National Flag increased this lack of confidence.

To us, therefore, who have wholly accepted the great ideals and the virtues of America, it seemed imperative to contribute whatever possible and true on behalf of that nation. This work is designed to serve this purpose. The writer has not been in the Soviet Union, but he has accumulated vast information about Soviet medicine in the course of almost half a century. That information was derived from literature, the Press, and from long contact with Russians and non-Russians. It has been derived from Communists and non-Communists who have been in Russia and the "Satellites". Finally, we have examined most recent Soviet sources coming from the evaluations on the occasion of the 40th anniversary of the October Revolution and the XXII Party Congress which was held in the Autumn of 1961.

All this was sufficient to compel the author to endeavor to publish this work under its present title.

Moreover, it became obligatory for him to attempt to reveal the very spirit of Soviet and American medicine. Fortunately the truth is very gratifying for the Americans and there is hope that it always will be so.

May 6, 1962   DR. GEORGE A. TABAKOV

TABLE OF CONTENTS

PART I

INTRODUCTION TO MEDICINE IN THE UNITED STATES AND THE SOVIET UNION

PREFACE

I have known Dr. George A. Tabakov since 1926, when I became the President of the American College then in Sofia, Bulgaria. From 1926 to 1942, I followed his career closely in Sofia, years during which he was building up his reputation as a respected and very active physician in Bulgaria. The declaration of war by Bulgaria forced me to leave that country and go to Turkey and only after the war was I able to follow again the work of Dr. Tabakov. Following the war and the seizure of power by the Communists his activities on behalf of freedom of speech, freedom of choice in his work, and freedom in medical research led to his arrest, trial and imprisonment by the Communist rulers of his country. After the cruel suffering inflicted upon him recorded elsewhere, he escaped from Bulgaria and eventually arrived in the United States where he has been able to establish himself as a practicing physician. Like all his friends I have been amazed by his pluck and determination to serve the cause of freedom by all the means in his power, and remaining most faithful to America.

The work entitled MEDICINE IN THE UNITED STATES AND THE SOVIET UNION which he has arranged to publish, represents a part of his magnificent effort to oppose and expose the whole system of Communism at every point within the range of his ability. His long and thorough training in medicine and his conflict

with the Communist system in its harshest aspect enable him to write with knowledge and authority in this
field of scientific inquiry.

FLOYD H. BLACK
President Emeritus, Robert College,
Istanbul, Turkey

INTRODUCTION

Medicine in the United States and the Soviet Union is a treatise that has grown out of deep and contrasting experiences. After Dr. Tabakov obtained his M.D. degree in 1933, he served as a government country doctor in Pordim, North Bulgaria, where he also acted as school physician at Dr. Haskell's People's University. At the end of this appointment, the government awarded him "for having organized, with indefatigable labor, devotion and self-denial, an exemplary country health service."

Then in Sofia, the capital, he specialized in Pediatrics and also soon became editor of a medical journal. Later he became editor-in-chief of "Contemporary Medicine", continuing until removed by the Communists in 1951 because of having "Americanized" the Journal.

Before and during World War II, he wrote many leading articles for pro-Western newspapers against Nazism, racism and Communism and befriending the Jewish people. Having founded and headed a hospital in Salonika to serve the 240,000 Bulgarian minority in the Aegean area (though it actually served everybody,) he received a Gold Medal from the Bulgarian Red Cross, and became a "Citizen of Honor" of the Bulgarian community.

When the Communists took over his country in 1944, he was demoted for he was known to be pro-American. He was under constant surveillance and later, after having been placed in charge of the Hospital for Infectious Diseases, was arrested in 1952, sentenced to death and held in chains awaiting execution. Thanks to his wife and numerous discreet pro-Americans who secured hundreds of names on petitions for his "pardon," his sentence was commuted to life imprisonment. After almost three years, due to a revision of the case, he was released as innocent. But in his shattered condition he fell under a street car and lost his legs. On a trip to Czechoslovakia for medical treatment, while passing through Jugoslavia, he and his wife escaped, going to Paris where his son had been sent a month earlier.

After eighteen months in France he was admitted to the United States. His acceptance of a call to open an office in a small town was certainly not prompted by the profit motive, but rather by his desire to serve and to express his gratitude to America. The Chamber of Commerce appointed him as head of a Community Improvement Committee, in which capacity he has worked with vigor, keeping many people busy in the program. In 1961, a Community Festival sponsored by this Committee was described by a metropolitan newspaper as a type of cultural program hitherto "unknown in northern Ohio." The proceeds from this Festival as well as from other campaigns were designated as reserve funds for what is Dr. Tabakov's primary objective (approved by the C.C.) — the eventual erection of a "House of Culture."

His greatest concern is about the advancing Communism. Too many of our leaders, in trying to act as Christians, believe and trust the Communists who are quick to take advantage of this "weakness" to push us back and to eventually "bury" us. These "super-Christians" along with the rest who are indifferent as to what is happening, are selling us out to the enemy. This study is a timely and concerned effort to set the record straight.

As one news writer exclaimed, it would take a volume to tell of the doctor's European successes and sufferings, and another to tell of the zeal and inspiration he has attempted to inject into this quiet community where he lives.

— ALVA W. KNOLL, M.A., B.D.

PART I

INTRODUCTION TO MEDICINE IN THE UNITED STATES AND THE SOVIET UNION

INTRODUCTION TO MEDICINE IN THE
UNITED STATES AND THE SOVIET UNION

For eighteen months I was on the staff of the Babies' and Children's Hospital, Western Reserve University, Cleveland, Ohio, U.S.A. The day I had to quit was really a sad one for me because I had to separate from an institution whose standard of medicine from purely a scientific, methodological and spiritual point of view was on an unbelievably high level. I felt indebted to all of those wonderful scientific workers and the rest of the people there.

I shall forever remain grateful to Drs. W. Wallace, S. Spector, A. Tucker, R. Wedgwood, L. Mathews and W. Weil, — B. & C. Hospital; to Drs. C. Beck and J. Ankeney from the Chest Surgery Dept. of Lakeside Hospital; to Dr. H. Tucker from the Dept. of Neurology; to Dr. R. Bolande from the Pathology Dept., and to all of the other doctors and scientists from the other departments of the University Hospitals and the Western Reserve University School of Medicine. The remarkable erudition of them all, their clinical experience, skill and methodology, and their highly academic spirit, nobleness and responsiveness to my grave troubles will ever be a source of inspiration to me. I recognize my obligation to all of them, to the American science of medicine and to this great American nation.

My first thought was to forward them a letter of gratitude and appreciation. But it happened that at that time the Soviet situation was becoming more acute and I had the opportunity of reading a number of articles by prominent Americans who had visited the Soviet Union in 1958, and after, and who were sharing their impressions of Soviet medicine, — Adm. Rickover's *Echoes on Soviet Education,* Dr. Milton Senn's (Yale University) description of his visit to the Soviet Union, the extraordinary article of Dr. Edward Teller, the father of the U.S. hydrogen bomb, concerning the prospects of the U.S. and USSR sciences, etc., etc.

The material I read was interesting and in some ways very accurate and useful. Generally it was written by people who had been in the USSR for a few days or weeks, were unaware of the Russian language and were relating information only relevant to some individual aspects of Soviet medicine and did not afford the American medical profession a completely beneficial picture of the medical reality behind the Iron Curtain. So I decided that it would be useful for me to attempt to reveal in fuller form this Soviet medicine which I have been closely following for many years. By doing so, I thought I could give the strongest expression of my appreciation of U.S. medicine and its masters, proving that generally it is far ahead of Russian medicine and that the latter can hardly catch up to U.S. medicine in the foreseeable future.

✿   ✿   ✿

From our predecessors we inherit in two forms the genetic traits characteristic of our race, people and parents, — the physical and the intellectual-moral heritage such as history, traditions, morals, ideals and virtues. To both of these, that is, to our organic evolution, according to G. G. Simpson, we owe our culture and our physical constitution. The intellectual-moral heritage, therefore, should not be excluded from our genetical nature on the one hand, and all that we are should not be attributed to the environment only, on the other hand.

If, consequently, we wish to usefully acquaint ourselves with Soviet medicine, science and their potentials in comparison with medicine and science in the United States, we have to know the underlying forces or drives characteristic of each of the two nations. In this respect they differ greatly. Take for instance, patriotism. It is far more zealously manifested by the Russian than the American. Or, to put it in another way, the American, being of a different genetical stock, geographical area and historical background, has outgrown the phase of patriotism felt by the Russian. In the American, patriotism is something kind, harmonized with the welfare and freedom of other people. For the American, it is something understood by itself, exists unnoticeably and would show only in case of extraordinary circumstances.

In the Russian, regardless of political regimes and cultural and intellectual level, patriotism is an ever active and dominating factor. If a young Asian goes to the Soviet Union, he will hear and read there such thoughts on nationalism and patriotism as he would never imagine if he were in the West. And in Russia this spirit is traced back five centuries, having been born first in the hearts of the earliest church fathers and tribal leaders. Following the formation of the Russian state, the Russian church was always progovernment, and while it worked under various forms such as Sacred Orthodox Church, or Slavic Orthodox

Brotherhood, it always enhanced the grandeur and the might of the Russian people, state and emperors. This is in sharp contradistinction from the Western church, Catholic and Protestant, which up to the present time and for centuries before have often been not only carrying on foreign policies of their own but fighting against the governments of their own countries, frequently disagreeing with respect to such issues as Communism, for instance.

Folklore bears the heavy imprint of patriotic grandiosity. Its most inspiring representatives are the epics by the name of byliny (past great events), chants singing the praise of immortal heroes, the greatest of which is Ilya Murometz, a powerful giant whose strength came from his contact with the earth. From this symbolization streams the peculiar Russian national romantic, idealistic and materialistic (realistic) philosophy of patriotism and might. The rich folklore simultaneously has served as an inspiration for the portrayal of its heroic characters in more realistic images by thousands of Russian writers and poets (*Taras Bulba* by N. Gogol, *Kazatsi and Hadji Murat* by L. Tolstoy, *Bogatiry* by M. Lermontov, etc.) and musicians (The opera *Sadko* by R. Korsakov, *Dobrinia Nikitich* by A. Grechaninov, *Men of Might* by A. Borodin, etc.) During the Stalin era, songs magnificent in gracefulness of melody, patriotic romanticism and meaning were produced.

Many of the common names, prior to the revolution bore the seal of the inborn Russian drive to feats of bravery, high patriotism and world power: Vladimir (Lord of the World), Branimir (protector of the World), Bcevolod (near to ruler-owner of all under the skies), Bogatir-Bogatirev (man of every great patriotic virtue), Bogdanov (one given by God), Lubomir (Lover of the World), etc.

Russian Narodnitsi (Populists) of the 19th century were the only exception to this uncomparable Russian chauvinism. But they are now forgotten and their spirit unknown to the new Russian generations. Thus anyone can conceive what all this means in the hands of a savagely dominating Communist ideology and Party and under an aggressive government like the Communist one in the USSR. This, in the long run, presents a tremendous challenge, — a moral rivalry for the West, and first of all for the United States.

We do not mean that the American people should become the type of patriots that the Russians are. We wish only to emphasize that the American is facing an immense force of competition, for which he has to compensate by developing and maintaining his overall capacities. Without feeling these things as they are, we cannot keep the superiority that American science now has over Soviet science, particularly in medicine, and we cannot survive.

BACKGROUND OF SOVIET MEDICINE HIGHLY PATRIOTIC AND MISSIONARY

Patriotism, often colored with romanticism and developing into chauvinism, underlies the best and the worst actions of many people throughout their history. A review of the past and present of all nations convinces us that all of them have had a "nationalistic" drive, but in the majority of cases they have followed a "reasonable" course. Usually this drive ultimately subsides. It never did in Russia. Facing the evolutionary trends which barred an open assault against the advance of freedom throughout the globe and made chauvinism and imperialism impossible, Russians found the new mask of Communism. Thanks to it, they succeeded in building the greatest single unified empire in world history. It is not difficult to guess what the future development will be. If Communism be ideologically unopposed by the free world, (I do not mean by war,) the next development will be not only an absolute political domination by Communism, it will be a new racial domination by the Russians over every other people on the globe. In the pursuit of these goals Russian medical science and Russian doctors play an active, vital and deliberate role. They claim that their motivation for this is their humanitarianism.

RUSSIAN INTELLECTUAL'S HIGH PATRIOTIC SPIRIT AND SENSE OF MISSION

M. V. Lomonossov, 1711-1765, who may very well be considered as the Russian Leonardo da Vinci, disputed with the German scientists concerning Russian history. "He was a great patriot . . . and he believed in the great future of his people."

D. I. Mendeleev, 1834-1907, a genius of chemistry and founder of the famous Mendeleev periodical system of chemical elements, fought Western spiritism and energetics and served Russian Tsarism.

N. V. Gogol, 1809-1852, is considered by some Russian and foreign literary experts as the greatest Russian classic writer. His epopee of *Taras Bulba* is impregnated with fascinating romanticism and patriotism. The first part of his masterpiece and greatest work *Dead Souls* ends with a passage not found in any of the geniuses of any nation or people.

"And, Russia, art not thou too flying onwards like a spirited troika that nothing can overtake? The road is smoking under thee, the bridges rumble, everything falls back and is left behind. The spectator stands still, struck dumb by the divine miracle: is it not a flash of lightning from heaven? What is the meaning of this terrifying onrush? What mysterious force is hidden in this troika, never seen before? . . . Russia, whither flyest thou? Answer . . . The ringing of the bells melts into music; the air, torn to shreds, whirls and rushes like the wind, everything there is on the earth is flying by, and the other states and nations, with looks askance, make way for her and draw aside."

F. Dostoevsky, 1821-1881, who, despite his anti-tsarism and painful Christianism, was the prophet of a peculiar Russian mystic world-wide missionary destination. He spoke to Russian multitudes with such a passion and sense of Russian historical humanitarian mission that people were falling on their knees and lamenting.

Count Leo N. Tolstoy, 1828-1910, the great Christian author of renown, — of *War and Peace, Anna Karenina* and many other immortal literary and philosophical works. In his essay, *On Shakespeare,* Tolstoy criticizes the great Briton from Lessing's like rules constituting the basis of true art. He accepts moderation or the so-called "realistic justice" as a fundamental prerequisite for anything to be a real work of art, and he denounces Shakespeare because of his lack of a sense of this artistic and realistic measure of moderation and justice. In support of this conception, Tolstoy cites examples from Shakespeare's works, mainly from *King Lear.*

Of course, this attack is not at all accepted by any of the Shakespearologists and men of literature, including even the falsifiers, — the Communists. But some explain this assault by Tolstoy as a result of jealousy about the immortal Briton, an attempt to dethrone him and thus place himself, a Russian, on the highest pedestal of world art geniuses.

THE GREAT PHYSIOLOGIST, — PAVLOV, A CHAUVINIST

I. P. Pavlov, 1849-1936. This man, as a result of the directives and orders of the Party, is the beginning and the end of Soviet medicine and biology. He is the mightiest means Communist despots use to survive the trend counterposed by the biological forces of freedom. This man was also not an alien to the trend of extreme patriotism, representing a sharp contrast to what one expects a great scientist, especially a physiologist, to be. He has committed himself outspokenly on the issue of patriotism. Here we are citing from one of Pavlov's pupil's (D. A. Birukov) biographical books honoring the great physiologist:

"Our country opens vast fields before our scientists . . . and we ought to repay it to the highest possible degree . . . I do not at all consider the German surgeons better than ours, and in no case would I agree to have a German operate on me . . . I cannot understand why they consider Paris as the Capital of the World. Our St. Petersburg (now Leningrad) is much prettier."

In 1927 while attending the 14th International Congress on Physiology, a cholelithiasis had disturbed him, requiring an urgent operation. It was suggested that he be operated on by one of the great European surgeons. Pavlov refused and was flown to Leningrad where he underwent operation by Prof. Martinov.

"I experience a feeling of excitement when I have to report before foreigners," wrote Pavlov. "Then you do, with incredible acuity, realize that you are a man — a Russian, that every bit of your labor benefits or damages your country."

He contemplated for a long, long time on what message to forward to Russian youth dedicated to science; his thoughts on this issue again showed the same super patriotic trend, — an all-round service to the native land. To a young Russian scientist on his departure to the United States for specialization, he said:

"In America there is nothing to learn in physiology. In respect to physiology, America herself is a student."

In 1935, the 15th International Congress of Physiology took place in Leningrad. There before the delegates, scientists of the whole world, he declared: "I am able to realize the grandeur of the war of liberation." What war of liberation and against whom Pavlov was speaking at that time remains obscure. It only reveals the mighty patriotic sentiments of this man. And what he was is a tradition in the history of Russian intellectuals.

SOVIET MEDICAL MEN — OPPORTUNISTIC AND DISHONEST AGENTS OF COMMUNIST IMPERIALISM

The servility of the Soviet academicians and doctor-scientists is shown in the following shameful phenomenon and crime, either by means of their participation in it or by their silence and therefore approval or lack of moral courage to oppose it.

The case we have in mind is the famous doctors' trial in Moscow which took place in 1952. About fifteen doctors, men and women, mostly of Jewish nationality, were involved through the accusation that they had been poisoning top Soviet functionaries whom they were treating. That the accused, imprisoned and tortured by means of medieval techniques and by the use of Pavlov's teaching, had indeed been doing the poisoning was surely "proved" by the participation of Communist academicians. The same barbarous methods and the same participation of the academicians were applied in the thirties against Dr. Kazakov, an endocrinologist who, with others, was accused of having poisoned Maxim Gorky, the great proletarian writer. Dr. Kazakov and his colleagues were all executed.

This shameful and barbarous event had repercussions in the "satellites" who virtually copy the Soviet "experience" and methods. There, also, a number of doctors were accused of espionage for the U.S., or for other Western countries and sentenced to death or to life in prison.

In July, 1950, the historical joint session of the USSR Academy of Sciences and the USSR Academy of Medical Sciences took place in Moscow. It was devoted to Pavlov's physiological teaching and its ingraining as the main basis of Soviet biological science. The most celebrated and outstanding Russian scientists were presented at this session. Also, a great number of guests from the Communist empire attended. Indeed Stalin was living, and watching what had been planned and what was going on. The "happy" scientists showed the most excessively humiliating servility that ever occurred in human history.

For under the terror of the emperors, the intellectuals like Belinsky, Herzen, Lavrov, Dobrolubov, Pissarev, Dostoevsky, Lermontov, Pushkin, and many others were all sentenced to death, deported to slave labor in Siberia or deep in the Provintsia, or imprisoned because of their resistance. But these "gentle" Communists, academicians, "fighters" for the welfare of the people and for freedom, those who are continuously repeating the names of the above heroes, wear, each of them, many medals, titles and awards of distinction by the most savage satrap — Stalin.

Telegrams and resolutions abounded in honor of Stalin, containing a most superfluous language of adoration and superlatives. Phrases such as the following were common:

"Dear Joseph Vissarionovich,

Together with the Soviet people, we are proud and endlessly happy that you are heading world progress and progressive science. We pledge to you, dear Comrade Stalin, to do our utmost. . . ."

"Long live our beloved teacher and leader . . . the great Stalin. . . ."

With such words and declarations the session was opened and closed.

At the opening, following the praises for the great Stalin and Pavlov, there were denunciations of Western science and scientists, especially of those of the United States. Third on the row were the "scapegoats" in the USSR. A number of them were denounced because they had deviated from Pavlov's lines. What those lines were, no one knew up to that moment, and no one knows them precisely today. The "scapegoats" were academicians L. A. Orbelli and I. S. Beritov, university professors P. S. Kupalov, P. K. Anokhin, Dr. Stern (a lady of Jewish nationality) and several others.

The sin of this lady was that she was a helpless woman of Jewish descent and had admitted the existence of cerebrospinal barrier interfering with the passage of various substances including the streptomycin and suggested the suboccipital injection of the antibiotic. Such an "individuality", "autonomism", under the nose of the almighty main brain cortex was a heresy and had to be denounced.

One may say that such was the epoch and those highest ranking scientists, in order to survive, had no other choice but to pay adoration to Stalin; that all this was not sincere in the least degree. This, however, is only partly true. Such moves, when preached by scientists in a country with a dictatorship, greatly impress the masses. The latter are generally very sensitive to the Russian national stereotype of extreme patriotism. And Soviet science and medicine, from the top to the remotest in Siberia, are developing under this force, deadly perilous for the rest of mankind.

The effect of such influences becomes evident when one recalls the evacuation of European Russia, or the epic battles in the winter of 1943-44 in the open fields of Kursk and Harkov. Tens of divisions of all sorts on both sides took part in these battles. The combat lasted several days. Three times each of those cities fell into enemy hands. With what the Germans and Russians showed there and at Stalingrad, anything else in history would seem like a joke. And again, there the Russians prevailed, the Russian muzhik, the same that destroyed Bonaparte. Why? Because the Russians had stronger patriotism ingrained within their very being in the course of centuries, including Stalin's reign. In a future war those people will fight with the same determination. This we all have to well remember.

No Difference Between Scientists of Stalin's and Khrushchev's Era

What was the attitude of the same Russian scientists following Stalin's death? 1957 was the 40th anniversary of the October Revolution. All of the Russian medical journals published numerous reviews devoted to the achievements in the field of medicine and public health. Their authors were Soviet men and women scientists, academicians, doctors, university professors, biologists and physiologists. *There was not a single word of praise, recognition or justice for the sake of Western medicine and especially for the great merits of American medical science.* For the basis of development and progress of Russian medicine is first of all American medical science. There were superfluous boasts, denunciations, falsifications and an attributing to themselves scientific merits belonging to Western scientists, representing old American or Western science as theirs, and new. Later on, in the course of this review, we will amply illustrate the dishonesty of the Russian scientists who are shameless opportunists, agents of Communist imperialism and slavery. Here now it will suffice to cite a few examples only.

1. Prof. M. A. Klebanoff is a well known phthisiologist in the West, who works in Kiev-Ukraine. In the Foreword to A. E. Rabukhin's book *Epidemiology and*

Prophylaxis of Tuberculosis, issued in its second edition on the occasion of the anniversary, Klebanoff writes:

"... the author takes a critical approach toward the unjustified optimism which some of the foreign authors show in evaluating the epidemiological status of tuberculosis in the capitalistic countries ... while the lethality there has abruptly fallen, the morbidity of tuberculosis has insignificantly decreased ... and because of that there are still a great number of tuberculous people — Japan, 3 million (1952); U.S., 1.2 million; German Federal Republic, 500,000 (1950);" etc.

Using those old statistics, unrelated to the population and to the era of PAS and Isoniazid which appeared just about that time, Dr. Rabukhin himself does not compare them with figures regarding tuberculosis in the Communist countries. The author and the reviewer show the same dishonesty, inobjectivity and servility.

2. In *Voproci Okhrani Materinstva i Detstva* (Problems of Protection of Motherhood and Childhood) the prominent Soviet infectionist, university professor, D. C. Futer, published (February 2, 1958) an exhaustive review on "The Status of Combat Against Polio in USSR." In discussing the prophylaxis and the possibility of successfully preventing the disease by means of vaccine, he mentions this all in virtually two lines! And it is the last sentence of the lengthy article, with the name of Salk being written in Russian letters. Why not? In USSR there are so many names of non-Slavic extraction that the 400,000 isolated physicians can

easily be fooled, especially when he does not mention the nationality of the scientist.

3.   The journal of *Pediatria* is issued in 42,000 copies and is spread throughout the Communist empire.   In the second (February) issue of 1959 there appeared a strange comment on the part of the editorial staff. This passage we here give in abbreviated form:

> "In Hiroshima on the occasion of Children's Day, May 5, 1958, was unveiled the monument dedicated to the children who were victims of the atomic bombs. . . . For ten years doctors have fought to save the life of the little Teico Sasaki. . . . Now she has died of radiation . . . , her death has shocked the entire Japanese nation."

Of course, it "shocked" also the "noble" Soviet academicians and doctors, though a little late — nine months following the event! Natural enough, for the moral nature of those scientists was for them to keep silent when the Hungarians and Tibetans were smashed by Russian or Chinese tanks or deported to Siberia or central China and buried there alive.

On the pretext that the Polish "reactionary" elements had undertaken an untimely uprising in Warsaw in 1944, Moscow Communists allowed thousands of the elite of the Polish patriots to be destroyed by the Nazis. The same Communists earlier in the Polish-Soviet war destroyed 11,000 innocent Polish officers only because they were future potential enemies of Moscow. On this and many other similar occasions the academicians did not protest but remained unmoved. But they shamelessly dare to blame, fifteen years later, the U.S. which was an ally of the forces against the Nazis and which gave vital help to the USSR for its survival.

Such is the moral standard of those disgraceful men of medical science of the USSR, members of the new class, privileged and guarded by the Party's cruelty and criminality. These examples of the hypocrisy of the USSR are the very ones to whom many American scientists are paying respect and becoming friends: G. N. Speranski, V. A. Vlassov, U. F. Dombrovskaia, M. C. Maslov, V. I. Molchanov, P. A. Ponomareva, M. A. Skvortsov, O. D. Sokolova-Ponomareva, A. F. Tour, I. V. Tsimbler and others. They are received abroad by the American scientists and are receiving the Americans visiting the USSR. They are also receiving all of the blessings of the Communist state, — high posts, high salaries, awards, distinctions and praises. In return they are repaying the Party dictatorship on every occasion by attacking especially the U.S., degrading its men of science and infecting the minds of the Soviet people with the meanest ideas about the American world. Their number hardly exceeds two to three hundred. The vast majority are neglected.

Their latest demonstrations of faithfulness and thanks to the government are reminiscent of those of the Stalin epoch. The doctor-scientists again now express their profoundest thanks to the Soviet government and personally to N. C. Khrushchev. (H.A.M.S. of USSR #9, 1961.) Here is what they now say regarding the latter leader:

"Exclusively valuable appears the application of the physico-chemical methods in biology which N. C. Khrushchev pointed out as early as at the

XXI Congress of the Communist Party of USSR."
(I. M. Maisky, *Herald of the Academy of Medical
Sciences of USSR,* #10, 1961.)

Comrade Khrushchev! He understands physico-chemical methods in biology as much as the devil understands the Holy Gospel! That the academicians are
instruments and agents of the Party is evidenced by
the following passage:

"The medical scientists are conscious of the
colossal significance of their labor for the cause of
the establishment of Communism. Greeting the
XXII Congress of the CPSU, we assure our native
Communist Party that we are ready to give all
our powers." (Leading editorial, *Herald of the
Academy of Medical Sciences of USSR,* #10,
1961.) The language is more restrained than that
of the Stalin era but not less haughty and dangerous.

Of course, behind the ideological fog, stands Russian
Communist imperialism, and those scientists see themselves in relation to the rest of the world in the position
of the ancient Romans, or of those of the dead epoch
of early British colonial adventures, or of the Nazi.
They went so far as to attribute to themselves historically established merits of non-Russians.

The rebaptizing of clinical entities and signs to the
names of Russians started years ago and is eagerly
continued by the AMS of the USSR. For example:

Filatov's Spots — for Koplik's Spots.
Botkin's Disease — for Infectious Hepatitis.
Urovskoy Disease — for Cushing-Boeck Disease.

> Sokolovsky-Bouillaud — for Bouillaud.
> Aschoff-Talalaevsky Granules — for Aschoff's
>   and so on.

The latest argument is with respect to the priority in the description of arteritis obliterans. It was mentioned first by the Italian, Benivenni (1507). Now the Soviet academicians claim that its clinical birth began in 1864 when a Russian surgeon, Schach Parmianz, (not of Russian extraction,) dedicated an article to it.

What is the Opinion of Intellectuals and Scientists Abroad Regarding Soviet Scientists?

This question is a general one; the answer, therefore, will be relevant to all the Soviet intellectuals and men of science, not exclusively to those dedicated to medicine. There are two categories of people cognizant of the qualities of Soviet scientists and intellectuals. The one category is represented by the various visitors who, in the majority of cases, in the course of a few weeks, use interpreters to try to learn something; then they claim that they have understood the truth and the nature of the springs of scientific progress in the USSR. These visitors are the ones who, on their return to the West and especially to the U.S., start lecturing, publishing articles and even writing books about the "marvelous" methods in pedagogics, surgery, psychiatry and public health; about the unusually rich culture and erudition of Russian people of science and art; about the great hospitality of the Russians and their determination for peace; etc. With rare exceptions these people add much to the success of the Communist propaganda of lies and boasts.

The second category consists of people who know

the Russian language well, have followed Russian science, including medicine, for decades, and who even know Russian scientists and their scientist friends in the satellites by personal contact in the course of lectures, scientific discussions, at patients' bedsides and by their original writings. The opinions which we next cite belong to this second category of persons.

Behind the Iron Curtain there have been featured for a decade or more the so-called *Months of Soviet Science and Friendship* with a particular satellite country. Groups of Soviet scientists of all disciplines, and always selected from among the best available, visit regularly every year the respective "satellite" country or countries for a month. In those countries they give well selected lectures; they visit various institutions, universities and faculties, hospitals and eminent local personalities of science and intellect. In those countries they are honored by means of big, "spontaneous" and noisy meetings and manifestations of "gratitude and respect" to the high ranking guests. At the same time such scientific celebrations are carried on between the satellite countries themselves. They also are represented by groups of selected men and women of science. So the satellite hosts have the opportunity to observe both the Russians and those from the other satellites as well, as the latter exchange views about the former (the Russians).

The author of this survey has attended numerous meetings and lectures of the Russians, starting from Prof. Chumakov, Director of the USSR Central Institute of Virusology, and ending with Prof. Winogradov. I never heard one original and new idea or thing from them, though they were in the role of counsellors and mentors. While lecturing, they first had to boast and

to praise the Party more than to teach science. They
went very deep only in the field of Pavlov's teaching
and the accomplishments of his physiology and its
reflection upon medicine and biology. Of course, for
them this was easy because in dealing with Pavlov's
teaching they could feel quite safe since much of it
could be presented as a philosophy obscure even to
the lecturers themselves. During those months of
celebration, every evening we doctors and the professors in other fields shared our impressions. There were
hardly two interesting lectures out of fifteen or twenty.
The tendency to exaggerate from the beginning to the
end was the outstanding feature of those lectures;
blame of Western and American science, and preaching Marxism and Dialectics predominated.

Friends of mine, — professors of Medicine and other
Faculties, and scientists of various fields, — clearly felt
that generally all of the Soviet scientists who came
every year to lecture were twenty years behind. Isolated
for decades behind the Iron Curtain and endowed by
the Party with "commanding posts" and obedient audi-
tors, the lecturers often appeared ludicrous in the eyes
of local scientists who had been well informed and
trained in the West, and who had acquired, first of all,
the quality of honesty. My countrymen, friends of
mine, scientists, having specialized in Germany, France,
Italy, Austria or England, the majority non-Communist
but objective and honest, maintained that their conversations with the scientist delegates from Hungary,
East Germany, Poland and Czechoslovakia had confirmed their own opinions regarding the indisputable
inferiority of the Russian scientists in the delegations
of friendship from the USSR. Their general opinion
contained two main elements, — one, that the USSR

delegations of scientists were preachers more of Communism and less of science, and the other that they were selling old science, dating twenty years back, as new and as their own. This evoked unanimous dissatisfaction among local scientists, — hosts who were bitterly ridiculing the Russians.

WHAT SCIENCE THE SOVIETS WERE SELLING ABROAD

There was a widely advertised and praised Soviet biologist, — a bacteriologist by the name of G. Boshian. His thesis was that every microbe has its viral form which was not virulent but which was transferable to its virulent microbial form. He claimed proof in that he had established this truth for the fifteen most pathogenic microbes. The Communist press strongly supported Boshian's progressive "findings" and the Communists were very proud of this new "confirmation" of the scientific reliability of dialectics. However, while Prof. Chumakov, a virusologist of renown and Director of the USSR Institute of Virusology in Moscow, was lecturing, he was asked what his opinion was regarding the claims of Boshian. He held him up to ridicule by saying that Boshian's claims would be true if an elephant could come out of a donkey or a head of cabbage out of a pumpkin seed. There were extensive comments about this in local medical and biological circles. In the course of years, Boshian, together with his "science," was forgotten everywhere.

Z. A. Lebedeva caused a sensation by her pathologoanatomical findings in 1952. She claimed that the primary complex is not the first organized form (earliest manifestation) but the focal one which is the pro-phase of all subsequent forms. These foci are formed concomitantly with the primary complex which, in fact, is nothing but a more prominent one. Thus the rest of the focal formations are not hematogenic spreading of the infection presented by this more prominent primary complex but the product of the same early invasive hematogenic dissemination. To this early hematogenic dissemination but not, or not only, to secondary disseminations, becoming active foci are attributed the so-called secondary infections or superinfections, endogenous not exogenous. By the same token, some Communist phthisiologists accept the existence of two or more primary complexes in one and the same person as a regularity, while Western scientists have described a very limited number. The theory and findings, if there are such, of Lebedeva appeared something very new in the old field of tuberculosis, a very attractive credit to the Soviet scientists. However, Z. A. Lebedeva's thesis was received coldly by the majority of the Soviet men of science; it was not confirmed by any of the leading pathologoanatomists, and some, from the very beginning, declared their doubts as to the authenticity of the claims and finally all was forgotten. Today I do not find a single reference to this unique discovery following Robert Koch's historical contribution half a century ago. While the scientists of the USSR were reserved regarding this discovery, those in the Satellites were eagerly basing their understanding of tuberculosis on it and were writing articles and books in conformity to it.

Here is one last example of Communist science, though in the field of plant biology. The Party needed abundance and speeded up production, especially of agricultural products. This depended not only on the spirit of the peasants, but also on the methods of

treatment of the soil. So in the USSR the method of
deep digging of the soil was widely advertised and
made obligatory. The presumed increased productivity in this case was linked, first of all, with the
improved soil biochemistry. Everywhere, therefore,
behind the Iron Curtain, this method of deep digging
was imposed. All who disagreed were bitterly and
mercilessly denounced by the vast majority of their
colleagues. In Bulgaria the old and highly respected
university professor of agriculture, by the name of
Stransky, became the "scapegoat." He was nearly
declared a people's enemy. By whom? Besides his
colleagues, by the president Cherventkov, a brutal
and maniacal ignorant Stalinist. Their side had to
share such an eminent and bold scientist in the medico-
biological field as Prof. M. Popoff, awarded by the
USSR Academy of Science for his contributions in
activation of plant growth and productivity. He was
an anti-racist and as ambassador to Germany during
Hitler's time, he resigned, refusing to agree with Nazi
racial concepts and pressure. This time he had to
obey and follow the general line! Such were the fruits
also of Michurin-Licenkoist selectionism in agriculture.
Meanwhile the corn in Bulgaria producing the heaviest
crop was American but under the innocent number of
29!

What happened later? Several years of failure followed, then all of the objections of the opponents of
this method proved true. Communists started to
cautiously retreat. The latter was carried on in a
most humiliating way for them and for all previously
praised scientists. A man of mediocrity and semi-
educated, by the name of Maltsev, working as an agricultural technician far from Moscow, came up with

the conclusion that deep digging of the soil "was not on all occasions" advantageous; that in most cases a more shallow digging brings about richer crops . . .

IMMIGRANTS WHO HAVE GRADUATED IN THE USSR NOT EQUAL TO DOCTORS TRAINED IN THE WEST OR IN THEIR HOMELAND

In 1944-45 in Bulgaria, about fifteen doctors came from the USSR. They were Communists who had received their medical education and experience with the Soviets in the course of fifteen to twenty years before. The majority I know personally or have followed closely their activities in our country. Only one or two equalled the doctors trained in Bulgaria or the Western graduates. However, for only one of them the local Communists provided unusual advertising as a scientist. He was a surgeon by the name of K. Stoyanov. One can judge him by this simple event. On the occasion of his successful and "unusual" repair of a scarred and severely constricted esophagus by means of transplantation of a portion of the bowel, he was praised in the press, not by other scientists and specialists, but by one of his lady technicians only, undoubtedly inspired by him.

As the Soviet army was occupying our homeland, those doctors, countrymen of ours who had gone to the USSR between 1923 and 1939, dropped the military uniform and without meeting any of the routine requirements or procedures, assumed the highest positions in the medical administrative hierarchy of the country. In the University, however, they could not make it so successfully. One of those Soviet graduates and an indoctrinated man became Rector and a professor of dermatology at the newly founded university in the second largest city of the country, Plovdiv (old map name, Philippopolis). His name was P. Kristanov. His affairs were widely commented on in all circles, including friends of ours and members of the faculty. As a specialist he was below the average, mediocre. As an administrator (rector) he was involved in a number of criminal affairs, one being a misuse of a large sum of government money, and had to be removed from the university post, — and punished? No. He became secretary of the Division of Medicine at the Bulgarian Academy of Sciences! Most curious was the fact that the Communists, to save face, gave his post by contest to young Dr. Bachvarov, a non-Communist, graduate of the Sofia Faculty of Medicine, with extensive post-graduate and specialty training at the Hamburg Institute of Tropical Medicine and in Strasbourgh with the famous dermatologist, Pautrier. Such an elevation in science of a Soviet man or of a Communist is typical of the USSR, it is the official policy. The Party's qualifications are considered first and this is and will continue to be a major handicap of Communist science.

Soviet Medical Cadres — Their Origin and Potentialities

The bulk of the leading medical personalities of the USSR belong to the pre-revolutionary generation and to the period immediately following the October Revolution. Starting with the late Prof. M. C. Maslov, the creator and leader of the Leningrad Scientific School of Pediatrics, and with Prof. K. M. Bikov, the most outstanding representative of Pavlov's teaching, and

finishing with the pathologoanatomists, Skvortsov and
Abrikossov and the specialist in clinical nutrition, Prof.
Pevzner, all are now from 65 to 75 years of age and
are denominators and masters of Soviet medicine and
related sciences. Some of them are indeed people of
talent and of medical vocation. Nevertheless, their
early incorporation in the foundations of Soviet medicine, the privileges with which the Party endowed
them and the great support by the Party regime of
medicine in general, have helped them to advance in
the hierarchy, to accumulate great experience and
knowledge and to secure for themselves an exclusive
role. All of the privileges, consisting of higher salaries,
holding of multiple posts, awards, access to foreign
literature, access to the world abroad, etc., went to
them. The fact that their country was isolated and
that they were unrivaled gave them the opportunity
easily to preach their medical culture and easily and
frequently to sell old knowledge in place of new. Their
greatest quality, however, was their industry and devotion.

The rest of the leading and privileged medical cadres
consist of younger men. They have the positions as
heads of hospitals, university or hospital professors,
and heads of numerous institutes. Regarding their
intellectual and professional qualifications, however,
we can precisely judge by two facts, — their origin and
their accomplishments. With respect to the latter,
we can state that besides the routine practical achievements in the field of public health, they have not
attained anything remarkable. This is relevant also
to the older generation.

With respect to the first question, the origin of the
younger medical cadres, we have to remember that

because of the doctors' poverty, very few gifted young men are attracted to the medical profession. Also, there is little free and biologically sound competitive selection to insure greater rights and advancement to the most capable. This latter condition is a rule. The opposite is the rule in the American medical cadres and it constitutes that creative basis to which American medicine owes its great achievements.

University students are recruited from high school and professional school graduates. The high school education under Communism has been a varying one; the conditions of admission have been precarious, conflicting, ever changing and quite deceptive, because the principle of privileged admission has been strongly maintained. Sons of kolhozniks and workers of merit, sons of local Party authorities and their friends account for the greater percentage of admissions to high schools and universities. There are numerous evening high schools and professional schools, where through primitive and privileged qualification, workers and Party functionaries become qualified to aspire to academic careers. There are special speed up high schools, designed to train the most reliable young men, workers, etc. All of their staffs are Communists. Some of these schools run two classes a "school year" of several months. On the other hand, there has always existed a rivalry between the provincial candidates and those of the big cities. The latter have always had easier access to the high schools and universities than the former because the higher Party officials live in the large cities. Far from the universities and their circles, far from big city culture and connections, provincial children, including those of the Communists, have been the greater losers in all contests. The only way to assure access to the universities appeared to be by having the higher marks, — the highest grade of high school certificates. So there was a deliberate and silent agreement between the school authorities and the parents, including Party members and local Party leaders, to give higher marks than the children actually deserve. These high marks not only insure the access of the children to the competition procedures in the universities, but thanks to various other privileges, it floats many of them directly in without actual contest. Another vital advantage of such proceedings by the provincial authorities is that all are safe from any blame and even from perilous responsibility to the Party in the fulfillment of the Party-government plans regarding the availability of a sufficient number of "well educated" children and young men for various specialties and schools.

In the Soviet press in the course of the years, one has had the opportunity to read many curious stories. For instance, high school boys and girls are enlisted in advance in various sections of Government and Party services, — in military, naval, professional and political schools. This is often done regardless of the wish or will of the youths. But even in cases where their will is respected, later if it is changed, it is not taken into consideration. So for the victim there begins a period of struggle and moral suffering which makes out of the young man or woman an incapacitated individual who can never acquire the proper shape.

Every year the number of candidates for the university is tremendous but the chance of admission is much smaller. A person's calling has little to do with it, much less personal qualifications. Disappointment is bitter and in order to calm parents and Party members, the Party orders an increase in the quota and this gives entrance to new youths regardless of their inferior capacities. All this is the "dough" that makes up Soviet science.

If one, therefore, takes into consideration what freedom, justice and vocation mean in human creativeness, especially if he has experienced these things personally, he can then judge that the qualities of Soviet cadres of medicine and their actual possibilities cannot but be inferior to those of free countries and especially to the United States.

These facts are relevant to the entire Soviet intelligentsia, to the entire intellectual cadres, not only in the medical field. We have, however, to recognize that these disadvantages are, to some extent, compensated for generally by the more augmented school programs and by the much greater magnitude of the population involved in education as compared with the U.S. The other superiority of the USSR is the incomparable eagerness and dedication of the youth to education. This has been historically true and is not solely conditioned by the complex methodology and nature of the Communist system in which adoration of science borders upon pathology.

MEDICAL TRAINING

Basically, the university education in the USSR is something of the "classical" sort, both before and after the revolution and as it always has been in France, Italy, Germany and Austria. Ten years ago British delegates were praising the Soviet system of medical education. Much more so do various observers of later years. The praises concerned the strong maintenance of the unity between the basic and the clinical sciences. There are 23,000 physicians (Vrachi) produced in the Soviets annually; while in the U.S. the annual production is 7,000.

We have to recognize that any program of education represents only one of the essential elements of training. No matter how good, if the other constituents involved in the make-up of the doctors are bad, the program cannot compensate for this. What are those other essential elements that do or do not contribute to the success of the training program in USSR?

1. *The subjects.* In the Soviet Union, one-third of them are of purely military and political nature: Historical and Dialectical Materialism, Political Economy (Marxian, of course), History of CPSU (Communist Party of the Soviet Union), Organization and Tactics of the Infantry, Organization and Tactics of the Medical Services in Time of War and Peace, Military and Field Surgery, Air Defense, Defense Against Poison Gases and the Atom Bomb, and Practice, in categorized groups, of Various Military Weapons and Machinery. All this the medical student, any university student and even the high school student, is obliged to study and know, for Communism needs, first of all, soldiers for the war which it is preparing to wage in order to conquer the world. However, students, even the Communist youth, resent this part of the program and do all they can to avoid or minimize participating.

2. *The cadres.* They are the basic, paramount factor. We have already commented on this. Several examples, however, will be useful, though they are not all from the medical field or from the USSR. We re-

sort to the latter because they reveal the real spirit of the Communist system.

Pravda, organ of the Communist Party of the USSR, published in the Spring of 1956, the story about the famous "Academy of Agriculture K. Timiriasev" in Moscow. The article was entitled "Academicians — Speeders" because of the favoritism of the Director of the Academy toward a number of students who thus have been able to graduate in half the regular time. Names were given of all, the characteristics of the director and the numerous relatives he had admitted to the payroll of the Academy. Similar examples were pointed out throughout the USSR. Such phenomena are not isolated. He who reads the Soviet press, including *Krokodil* and *Literaturnaya Gazetta* knows what bureaucratism, favoritism and protection mean in Russia and what their magnitude is, and it all is implanted in the Satellites as an inevitable part of the Communist system.

In Sofia, non-Communist professors, including those of the medical faculty, continuously complained of the pressure upon them. The pressure was applied by Party functionaries. The professors were informed that certain students had to pass, or that they were to be re-examined three days after they had failed! They received threatening letters from students who had failed, or from their protectors. Finally they would receive telephone calls for the same purpose. Some students, as Communists, make the threats themselves, while others commit intimidation behind the mask of being Communist though they are not. This all unveils the possibilities of the Communist regime. One evening Professor B., *The Tiger at the Doors of the Polytechnic*, told us the following story: (He was of a giant-like build, a very gifted mathematician, a really tough character and horribly anti-Communist.) He had received an anonymous threatening letter from one of his students. At his next lecture he said, "One of my students sent me a letter, threatening that I'll be beaten. Well," he went on, "we are seven brothers and I am the youngest and the weakest. Nevertheless I'll not run away if it happens that this gentleman, or these gentlemen, decide to meet me somewhere."

Why are these things done? This is the way the Party can recruit faithful cadres; it cannot exist otherwise. For among the various forms of favoritism, such things encourage the students, the Party members. At other times another course is followed. In order to decrease the number of the competitors, or to divert students to other sectors of education or to industry, confidential orders may come from the ministry that 75% of them are to fail. Who would they be? Anyone except those protected by the Party. So double harm is done to the education. This is a regular practice followed by the regime when it wishes to turn the young people along predetermined lines.

One day in 1956, Miss X, a university student and daughter of writer Y (one of the most outstanding intellectuals of Bulgaria [non-Communist]), came to my office as a very dear friend. I had been her doctor since her infancy. She was extremely excited, and said to me: "Today our professor (a Communist in the University) interrupted his lecture and told one of the students to go to the blackboard and write one of the Latin terms he mentioned. This the student was unable to do because he did not know well the Latin alphabet. Angered, the professor called a second and a third student who showed the same ignorance.

The professor became so furious that he bitterly denounced them as 'the speeders' who were 'sitting on benches that belonged to the gifted youths who were at this moment working on the constructions'." All those that failed were privileged ones, "speeders," products of the high schools for privileged young men and workers. Their number is great. It increases because the Party aims at completely eliminating all "doubtful" elements who do not belong to the working class. And this is in Bulgaria, whose culture and traditions are on a higher level than those of the USSR. The present situation in the latter is nothing but the successor to the previous conditions described by the Russian classics as unprecedented in human society. This is a Soviet pattern copied.

With respect to favoritism, bureaucracy, injustice and unlawfulness we wish to unveil two examples which are typical of the Party members, who are of the opinion, as a new class that they are allowed to do anything for their welfare.

A Communist, director of a cooperative farm, started to build a private house for himself but lacked enough wooden beams. One night he called a number of his subordinates, who on his order tore down the farm library in the mid-village and carried the beams to the director's house. In the morning the peasants were unable to recognize their village because the structure, which had been of greatest distinction in the village, was missing.

One of the ministries obtained budget sums for a new experimental institution far from Moscow. Reliable friends and Party men were appointed director, dispatchers, experts, etc., to carry on the work of the institution. The gentlemen regularly reported about the course of the things on the spot and money they had drawn regularly in the name of the new institution. Inspectors from the ministry had been appointed to see the way things were going and reports had been submitted that all was going perfectly well. In the fourth year of the "foundation" of the "new experimental institute" a serious inspector had dropped in. At the location of the institute there was nothing of that kind. There was not a trace of any building, of any construction!

Post Graduate Training

In the USSR Post Graduate Training is carried on by the so-called Institutes for Perfection of the Physicians. There is a central one in Moscow and a dozen others throughout the USSR (Leningrad, Kiev, Khazan and others). They are of a more advanced standard, well equipped and possessing divisions of all medical specialties. Doctors come in groups and are instructed by highly qualified personnel. Each course lasts six months. Only doctors that are pointed out by their chiefs and the Party and under a certain age, have access to this type of training. Their number is limited but the flow is continuous and this contributes to the elevation of the standard of the USSR Vrach. This type of training and the confinement in work to one and the same field, presents the "specialization", and compared with that in the U.S., it is very inadequate. For in the latter country besides the many years of real specialization, there is an abundant literature, the prosperity of the doctor, the competition, the existence of permanent courses, even by mail, in the special fields of the doctor's interest to promote the creation of very highly prepared specialists. The same appraisal is valid regarding the U.S. medical student who, having entered medicine because of an internal drive, and sometimes despite poverty, works hard to achieve success in his chosen field. Says Dr. Y and his wife — both doctors who have escaped from behind the Iron Curtain, and we are citing both: "Communists say that there is no medicine in the U.S. but laboratory and techniques, no need of knowledge. But when we came here and saw what American doctors young and old know, and the way they apply it, we got shocked, so superior it was."

Some General Characteristics of Soviet Men of Medicine and Their Writings

The forewords of books, the leading articles of the journals, the reviews of Western sciences and of medical societies, echoes of international Congresses, even on any Soviet achievement of any nature, — anything on which they write, — all have an open ideological nature and spirit of servility to the bosses.

After praising the Party for its plan to create the Paradise on earth in the next twenty years, we find such echoes on the part of the academicians:

"Soviet scientist-doctors recognize the great significance of their labor for the cause of building Communism. Welcoming the XXII Congress of CPSU (Communist Party of the Soviet Union) we assure our Fatherland's Communist Party that we will give all our powers and knowledge . . ." (On the Forthcoming XXII Congress of CPSU — a leading article, *Herald of the Academy of Medical Sciences of USSR*, #10, 1961.)

"Scientist-doctors (not mere doctors, but scientists, — Author's Note) ought to make full use of the colossal possibilities provided for them in order to carry Soviet medical science toward new horizons. No doubt the workers in the field of protection of Motherhood and Childhood of the Russian Federation will do their utmost to successfully fulfill the tasks pointed out in the Program of CPSU." (A leading editorial in the *Problems of Protection of Motherhood and Childhood*, #10, 1961.)

Servility to the bosses is now as it was in the era of Stalin when he was pronounced by the same academicians "the Greatest Etymologist-Dialectician of all times."

"The application of the physico-chemical methods in biology appears especially valuable as Nikita C. Khrushchev pointed out as early as at the time of the XXI Congress of CPSU.

"In the report of Nikita C. Khrushchev at the XXI Congress of the CPSU, the significance of biology as the theoretical basis of medicine was demonstrated with exceptional perspicaciousness." (I. N. Maisky, *Herald of the Academy of Medical Sciences of USSR*, #9, 1961.)

Their praises of Communist doctor-scientists or of Communist medical science, their denunciation of the West and especially of the U.S., their boasts, all are expressed in superlatives: "Very great," "Immense contribution," "Great feat," "Greatest son of our Fatherland," "The pride of our science and country," "Most outstanding," "A most ardent

enemy," "A gangster," "A profoundly sworn people's enemy," "Highly genial," "The greatest scientist," and so on and so on.

A Poor Doctor Cannot Be A Good Doctor
and Soviet Doctors Are Poor People

Classical medicine was not created in laboratories
or institutions. Hippocrates, Galenus, Koch and Laenec
did not have them. First of all, medicine, medical
science and progress are products of the labor, observations and imagination of the vast majority of doctors. A great clinician by the name of V. Mollov
maintained that a poor doctor cannot be a good
doctor (in the broadest, scientific sense). Then, can
a Soviet doctor be a good doctor when he is a poor
man? Science and scientific progress are inconsistent
with poverty. A French classic once said, "If some
day private property is abolished, the greatest poverty
on earth will take place." And poverty and ignorance
go together, and in the USSR there is no private
property, no prosperity.

A fundamental requisite for an outstanding doctor-
ship is the welfare of the doctor, starting from the
early years of his training and practice. The availability to the doctor of the widest facilities, means for
continuous post graduate education, economic security,
political freedom and even rest of a sufficient degree,
is of paramount significance. How can this indispensable element be realized by the Soviet doctors?
How is its lack reflecting upon the doctors' morals
and activities? It is a tragic truth that the Soviet
doctor has nothing. Even his professional skill does
not belong to him, but to the Communist society, of

course.   Generally the Soviet doctor is a hard working slave.

First, the physician in the USSR was deprived of
the title of "Doctor."   They endowed him with the
honor of being called Vrach.   That is a sort of semi-
physician.   The titles of real honor are secured only
for those who are blessed by the Party, obedient to it
and in rare cases, because of extraordinary ability.
So the titles they have are: Junior Scientific Worker;
Senior Scientific Worker; Candidate of Medical Sciences; Doctor of Medical Sciences; Professor-Doctor;
Correspondent of the Academy of Med. Sc., Member
Correspondent of AMS.; Doctor-Member of AMS. and
of the Soviet Academy of Sciences; Scientific Worker
of Merit; etc.

Those titles are not only a sign of scientific distinction, but of pay as well.   For while the ordinary physician, "Vrach" has an average monthly pay of a
semi-specialized factory worker, that is, 600-700 old
roubles, the Junior Scientific Worker gets 200 roubles
more, the Senior Scientific Worker 350 roubles more
and so on.   The academicians and professors are paid
very high salaries, between 1500 and 2000 roubles.
And as a rule, every one of them has several additional
posts for which they are paid!   So the fight is, at least,
not for science per se, but for the pay because the
basic salary is insufficient for the doctor to meet his
most trivial needs and those of his family.   Of the
nearly 400,000 physicians, about 90% are of the lowest
category.   By all this the Party aims at keeping the
obedience of the majority by privileges for the small
minority.

The Soviet Vrach has no right to the choice of a
job, place of job or residency, or of changing his job

or preference. He can start specialization or post-graduate courses and education, only if he is endorsed by his chief in consultation with the Party authorities. To go abroad is a dream for him which he can never realize, as it is only the privilege of the coryphaei who are backed by the Party. He can only hope to visit some of the Communist countries.

The Soviet physician is one of the most criticized servants of the society, held responsible for anything which patients think he is guilty of. He is always wrong. Patients are categorized and in this order served at the clinics and hospitals. The workers are in the first category. Then the workers themselves are categorized, the miners being first in the row. And as the doctor has to take into consideration many factors, something flexible by itself, complaints are made against him.

At his place of work if he is some sort of chief, the doctor has to give an account to the Party bureau as to what he is doing and why. He is also obligated to attend numerous meeting each day or week. These meetings have a devastating effect upon the spirit of Soviet citizens. This led their poet of revolution, V. Mayakovsky, to dedicate a sarcastic masterpiece of his to these crucifying meetings. If the doctor is OD and is visited by a lady, even a colleague, he is suspected of immorality (if he is not a Communist) and is "invited" by the Party Secretary to explain and is advised to be careful. If he is very polite with patients, not workers, he again is characterized and blamed for bourgeoise manners. Naturally he is hurt, seeing the difference between himself and a colleague who is privileged because of his membership in the Party. This, as well as the poverty, makes him a creature unwilling and incapable of being interested enough in science. The Soviet Vrach is an unfortunate worker, exhausted by responsibilities, long working hours, paper work, fear and poverty.

He does not have enough money to pay the subscription of even one Russian journal. This is evidenced by the small number of medical journals printed in comparison with the great number of physicians. As to his access to foreign literature, especially current, there is nothing which can help him. He has no right to privately subscribe and he can make very little use of the one or few foreign (Western) journals received only by libraries and some institutions of the largest cities. If he finds them available, he is obligated to use them on the spot. Any American or Westerner, therefore, can imagine the extent to which the Central Reference Journal, containing very brief summaries of current foreign medical publications, can be useful to the doctor. This is a journal that appeared several years ago through which the Soviets are attempting to compensate for the lack of hundreds of current Western publications.

Finally, the Soviet doctor has no freedom of initiative. All he does has to be planned and is controlled by the local authorities of the Party or by the professionals, Communists, organized at a particular institution.

From what was said about the Soviet doctor recruited from the middle schools, we can draw the following conclusions with respect to their possibilities in the future.

1. The Soviet school system is richer than the American, but it is also influenced by political material, favoritism, limited horizons and superfluous theoriza-

tion. The same is true of the Soviet physicians. They are socially underestimated, politically dependent on the Party, poor people, and scientifically backward because of narrow education. This accounts for their sterility in the field of imagination and scientific medical progress. To survive they have to contrive to boast much and even to lie.

2. However, in the long run, the above handicaps will be more or less compensated for by the unprecedented government support of education and by the gifted youth, eager to learn; by having almost an ingrained drive to learning along the classical lines; by the very large number of youth and people involved in education, research and science. From a bio-social point of view, this latter point is very likely to result in the production of extraordinary cadres in all fields of medicine. The only factor hindering such a possibility is the lack of freedom which is essential to the working of the biological laws in human society or in the individual, and which is the greatest creative factor.

Remarkable Medical Books in the USSR

There are at present three publications which are a unique feat of USSR medicine.

1. *Bolshaya Meditsinskaya Encyclopedia* (Grand Medical Encyclopedia). It was started in the early thirties and completed before World War II in over thirty volumes, though smaller and with less contents on each page than the well known *Encyclopedia Brittanica*. Currently it is appearing in its second edition, coming twenty years after the first. This edition is in thirty-five volumes, with 100,000 copies (the

former had 21,000) and up to the present twenty-one volumes are out of print.   In the first edition 1718 authors and 183 editors participated while in the second edition, in its twenty-one volumes which are out of print, at this moment 2500 authors and 642 editors have taken part.   The editor-in-chief of the new edition is the academician Prof. A. N. Bakulev, the famous heart-chest surgeon.   Because in one sense this publication appears to be a real scientific feat, though of a badly Communist character, we should give some more information as found in Soviet sources, and relevant to the scientific value of the work.

Section on Internal Diseases

1.   The indications of the corticosteroids are not given with sufficient clarity.

2.   Heart arrhythmias — the new chapter is worse than the one in the first edition.

3.   Agralunocytosis — one gets the impression that any drug can cause it.   The white hemogram is not clearly given.

4.   Addison's Disease — the term of breast nipples is used instead of areolae mammae where this latter term means charm, fascination, radiancy, etc.

5.   Jaundice — it is claimed that itching accompanies the obstructive type only.

6.   In the DD of the hemolytic type of jaundice nothing is mentioned about the hemolysis in this illness and its degree, as well as of finding urobilin in the stools.

7.   Aldose is mentioned in the DD and nothing is said regarding the other ferments, and first of all, of the transaminase.

8.   The functional diagnosis of liver pathology is

insufficiently described, especially the physiological tests.

9.   Nothing is mentioned concerning the treatment of the antiagglutinins with corticosteroids.

10.   To patients suffering from Infectious Hepatitis, drinking large amounts of mineral water is recommended.

11.   Very little is said regarding the indications and prescription of antibiotics.

Many other defects are found and much unscientific information is given also.

Volume on Pediatrics

Among infectious patients whose isolation is obligatory by law, the isolation of diphtheria, poliomyelitis and meningococcal meningitis patients is not mentioned at all.

Pertussis and Poliomyelitis are excluded as diseases against which effective immunization exists.

(A number of other mistakes and inaccuracies are mentioned — Author's Note.)

Section on Endocrinology

To this theme 46 articles are dedicated. As defects, the following are pointed out.

A series of articles are not exhaustive, lack clarity and in many instances are inaccurate.

In the article "Antithyroid means" the very important question of their clinical application is missed.

The articles on "Basedow's Disease" are of obviously surgical trend for the sake of other aspects of the treatment; there are also a number of defects. For instance, nothing is mentioned with respect to the application of the corticosteroids in thyreotoxicosis.

The information relevant to the application of the radioactive Iodine in Basedow's Disease is wrongly given.

The author brings out the old view of Todd, which nobody shares today, on the possibility of a carcenogenic effect on the part of 1^{131}.

He says that the surgical treatment of Basedow's Disease is indicated, especially when exophthalmos appears. This is not true because exophthalmos does not always coincide with the degree of damage of the organism . . . It is known that sometimes following operation and the thyreotoxicosis subsides, exophthalmos appears.

The chapter on "Hypergenitalism" is wrongly written . . . the terms of hypergenitalism and the Pellizzi syndrome are confused.

(The above remarks regarding the defects of the three specialties are given in the article of Prof. N. Nishereshevsky, *Clinical Medicine*, #10, 1961, Moscow.)

The reader can conclude for himself as to what this huge publication would look like when he takes into consideration the ideological factor and the slavery under the Communist Party. In the present rapid and dramatically progressing medical science, one gets the definite impression that it was less for the sake of usefulness and more for remunerative purposes, and last, for ascribing the Communist seal to science in the broadest sense of the term, that made the Communists produce this otherwise magnificent work.

2. *The Medical Experience of the Great Fatherland War, 1941-1945.* This is a kind of Encyclopedia relevant only to the war period experience on the battlefield and in the rear. It consists of eighteen vol-

umes the size of the *Bolshaya Meditsinskaya Encyclopedia,* and is written by many contributors, — participants in the war. This publication, again, impresses the foreigner more as an extraordinary accomplishment and as a proof of the esteem of learning, than as a scientific work of lasting duration and usefulness. It also is contemplated to serve in a future war.

3. *An Atlas of the Main Brain Cortex of Man.* This publication appeared in 1955. It is a great accomplishment by numerous authors (neuropathologists) under the editorship of the Soviet's most outstanding neurologist (Armenian descent,) C. A. Sarkissov; price, 75.5 old roubles.

It is well to point out here the most characteristic features of Soviet medical books:

a. They are all based on Pavlov's teaching of Nervism, and on Marxist-Leninism.

b. All of them unsparingly emphasize the grandeur of Russian medicine and science in general.

c. All are extremely accessible to the foreign reader because of the very low cost. For this reason they are widely bought in the West, especially in the countries now under Communist yoke. In the latter the most frequently seen stores are the book stores, and those selling Russian literature are overcrowded. There one can find most interesting books at fantastically low prices. Even in Paris, in the few "Russian" book stores, the visitor may see an unbelievable variety of Russian works on political as well as non-political themes, interesting for men of every race, nationality and profession.

At the same time, because of their high price and the currency restrictions, Western medical books are but a dream for the doctor behind the Iron Curtain.

In this manner Communist regimes confine the doctor's interests to the Fatherland's sources alone. If to this one adds the fear of citation of foreign authors, the picture is completed as to the professional-scientific scope of the physician in the Communist empire. The few Western books found in the libraries can never meet the everyday needs and interests of hundreds of thousands of doctors. This forced "isolationism" is one of the reasons that every one of the coryphaei of Soviet medicine is talkative, to be in the position of being a revealer of the "great" science, either as his own or as of his country, when relaying information he has read in some Western publication.

PUBLICATION OF MEDICAL BOOKS

For years following the October Revolution, there were almost no original Russian books and the Communist regime and scientists had to use available foreign ones including those published by the contra-revolutionary Russians who reached Western Europe, especially Germany. There was a remarkable House in Berlin which published in Russian the best Western medical works. At the same time the Bolsheviks were translating Western classical books of medicine as well as gradually producing their own. Of course, they did not recognize any international laws of authorship, and never paid a penny to the authors whose works they translated and reprinted. "All belongs to the people, people are one throughout the globe, and since we are the people and working for the people, all we take is our right." An increasing number of collective works are published annually by institutions, hospitals and organizations. In the vast majority of cases, the volumes are rather small, 150-350 pages. The same is true of about ninety percent of the textbooks. They rarely exceed 400 pages of the ordinary format. The circulation varies, the average being from three to five thousand; rarely it is from twenty to fifty thousand. Authors are paid for the amount and nature of work and not according to the circulation. Royalties are very good and of three categories.

As to the publication itself it is sometimes very painful for the author. If a doctor decides to write a book, first, he has to give preference to the Russian national sources and if he intends to use foreign ones, that is, first of all American, he has to, by all means, do this in such a way as to discredit Bourgeoise science and praise the Russian. Second, he has the moral right to use Western data and knowledge without citing it, that is, he can freely plagiarize and attribute all merit only to Soviet science. Third, regardless of the nature of the work, he has to pay tribute to the Party, its gods and philosophy. The manuscript then is submitted to the Director of the Government Editorship.

He himself passes it to the recensionists in the field the author is dealing with. These recensionists are generally two or three in number. As a rule they are reliable Communists so that, later on, if there is something wrong with the published work, the chief editor is able to defend himself. This checkup of the works by the specialists takes months and as a rule, they also make recommendations which the author ought to take into consideration. This may be repeated several times.

Suppose the work has ultimately been brought to the point of readiness for publication; the Director may declare that since the book was not planned in advance, the author must wait for his book to be included in the next year's plan. It is true that they have to have some room for "outstanding" works which were not planned for in advance, but you never know what the situation is and what criteria are used. In such cases the author has two ways left, (1) to use the support of mighty personalities, if he has such, or (2) to try in one way or another to bribe the director or some of his assistants or some of the recensionists. Sharing part of the royalties is widely practiced. This also helps secure a better classification of the book and better royalties.

The extent to which works may be damaged is evidenced by the following example: Late one evening in 1952, I visited Professor X, one of the highest scientists and experts in our country in his field. I found my friend reading a newly published Russian book of his specialty. His opinion of Russian scientific literature was that hardly five out of a hundred are remarkable in any sense. So I was greatly surprised when he told me that this is one of the few good Russian works. Then in 1956 many Soviet scientists visited our country. This attracted our attention to the Russians again. My friend, the professor, was, and is, a determined anti-Communist, but they keep him because they desperately need him. He shared with me his impressions and those of his colleagues concerning the Soviet guest lecturers. Ninety percent of the feelings were negative. I asked him whether the aforementioned scientist was one of the guests.

"No," he said, "but wait; I have something else very interesting to tell you. One of the visitors from the USSR in our field is the director of one of the institutes of Stalingrad." (sic, now Volgagrad!) "This man im-

presses us all as one of the Communist science mediocrity. When I raised the question about the outstanding book I read three years ago, and its author, the
Communist director replied, 'Yes, I know him very
well and his writings as well. I was chief recensionist
of his first work and I had to remove considerable portions'."

Professor X continued, "Now you see what this savage man has done and why I felt that there was something puzzling in the book which, anyhow, delighted
me so much when I first read it."

The Soviet press abounds with reports and complaints about such abuses, bribery, protectionism, slowness and strange hostility to some authors and lack of
response to the just cause of others.

As we have already mentioned, publishing work of
any kind is a government monopoly. The publishing
organization is called "GOSIZDAT" and the medical section "GOSMEDIZDAT." However, not all is concentrated
in Moscow where the chief "Union" government is.
There are branches of this central government publishing organization, for instance, in Leningrad, Kiev,
Lwov, and others. And as all is based on grounds of
political competition, planning, control by the Party
and poverty, one can image what confusion, injustice
and irresponsibility is engendered. On the one hand
everything is excessively delayed. On the other hand,
there is so much triviality being published. For the
authors must produce something in order to contribute
to the building up of local Communist authority and
"pride". The local Party organs have to concentrate
on fulfilling the plans; also to fight poverty of authors
and their own. If accused of overlooking, they emerge
safely because there are so many factors involved in

the matter and at the same time they can claim, in fact, they so act as having thought of encouraging new forces, ideas and science. Every new edition bears changes imposed by mad-partisan criticism in the press, meetings or personal "suggestions" by Party functionaries.

As to the delay of the books coming into existence, it is evidenced by the information contained in the very publications themselves. Their first pages show the date when the manuscript was submitted for print and also when it was published. The average period of time between the two is at least six months. The time spent while the work was in the process of endorsement and the time for distribution of the book is not mentioned. However, altogether, from the moment of the submission of the work to the government publishing house to the moment of its reaching the readers, at least twelve to eighteen months elapse! What a notorious fact that is, everyone can judge who knows the present fast development of science.

Following the publication of a book, regardless of its nature, it is subjected to public or to closed scientific circle discussions. If it is found that there is something "wrong" in the work, the author is openly advised to correct himself. Pasternak experienced this in the literary field, as have many others. Sometimes the book is withdrawn shortly after appearing on the market because of the incrimination of some part of the contents.

I'll cite here several examples, not all from the medical field or from the USSR. But the reader should know that at every institution in the "satellite" countries, there are Soviet "counsellors" whose appearance alone would make your hair stand up straight. They are following Soviet patterns in the countries to which they are assigned.

In 1955, a Soviet etymologist published a work on a number of words in the Russian language of obscure origin. One of these words was BOOZOOLOOK. He explained its origin thus. Centuries ago Russian border guards had to live at the very borders in settlements, together with their wives and children. So the residents of such a village-guard had been visited by people of another border village. The hosts had entertained the guests by serving them BOOZAH and LOOK, the former a kind of sour drink prepared from fermented flour, and the latter, leeks. These are the poorest things one can imagine offering to his guests. Though the story was relevant to the epoch of the emperors, it was humiliating for the Russian Communist dignity. On this occasion, *Pravda*, the Party organ, became infuriated and pronounced the author guilty of stupid research and etymology.

The post-revolution humorist, Michail Zhoshchenko, whose critical, humorous writings about Soviet realities created for him unprecedented popularity in the thirties, was forbidden to write and was sent to a concentration camp. Shortly after he reappeared in the early fifties and attempted writing in the manner of "socialistic realism" he died.

One of the most humanistic works before the October Revolution was *Sketches of a (Country) Doctor* by Dr. V. Veressayev. It was written in, let us say, a Tolstoyan manner and, therefore, different from the works of Axel Munte (St. Michael), Paul de Kruif and others. The same Veressayev wrote a second book relevant to the events of the very October Revolution. Its title was *The Impasse*, (V Tupiké, in Russian).

It was published in USSR and translated into Bulgarian. In 1945, the Communists took over in Bulgaria and the book gradually disappeared. Because at this phase when much of the savagery described in the book and attributed to the very revolution was still going on in Russia and now was beginning in Bulgaria with the enslavement by means of Russian force, the book was no credit to the regime and therefore was withdrawn and banned from libraries or bookstores. As friends were going to USSR for various reasons, I asked them to bring me a copy of the Russian edition. Every time I was told that it was impossible to find it.

After the Communists took over in Bulgaria, their foremost writer at that time, Orlin Vassilev, published a book entitled *The Resistance*. There it was stressed that the air raids over the country by the Anglo-Americans were following information provided to them by the Communists. Some of those Communist agents and apparatus were parachuted from USSR or landed by submarines. They could not use other than Russian equipment. This was especially compromising for the Communists mostly when they started the cold war by openly accusing the Americans for ruining our beautiful capital, Sofia. (It was "dirty" before the Communists came into power.) The book which had tremendous success and circulation was withdrawn only because of these passages. The author became richer than any other writer and somewhat bold, — he did not agree to "rewrite" the story. This still more boosted the interest in the book. People were paying fantastic sums on the black market to get copies stolen by the Communists and sold. These are the practices "the Satellites" learned from the Soviets where history, science, truth, written today, tomorrow may be reversed and on the next day be brought to the previous state. Such is the fate of man and anything he says, plans or does in the USSR.

This is precipitated either by the Party whose attitudes are unpredictable or from the "people." The latter way operates thus: Following the publication of a book, meetings, many of them at various parts of the country, take place. There an evaluation is made by the "people," public infested by mad Communists, — with the author answering. He thus is often bitterly denounced for his "deviations" and advised to make the necessary corrections in the second edition. At other times before the book is published it is discussed by the writer's secretariat or presidium or by a special committee dominated by Communists. It is subjected to the same processing in various collectives again dominated by savage Communists. Following such agony the author is "softened" to the point of either meeting the conditions put by the incompetent, jealous, savage "people" or having his book go unpublished. When a book has escaped this last procedure, it is brought on the Party line tracks by the Government publishing house.

A Polish doctor who has recently fled Communist Poland told me that the creation of a book or article behind the Iron Curtain takes place in this manner:

1. You reason that if you wish to have a success and put forth a new idea you have to turn to American or Western sources.

2. This means big, big trouble for you. So you have either to refrain from writing anything, as many prefer

not to commit themselves because they may get in trouble in the future, or to write something that would be "irreproachable." But this is not science, this is not creatively gratifying and inspiring to the author. These considerations hold in the selection of thematics in research and in its pursuit. We do not have, therefore, to wonder why Soviet medical science is lagging.

As to the number of books published annually, one can judge by the fact that in the year 1958-1959, 6,250 books in 32 major medical fields were published in the U.S., while six times fewer books were printed in the USSR.

SOVIET MEDICAL PUBLICATIONS AND THEIR COST

Some claim that Russian books are unbelievably low priced. This is only true about the books sold in the Satellites and other places outside the Soviet Union. In the Satellites, Russian books are sold at a negligible price that does not even pay for the beautiful binding. The unusually low cost is for the sake of the satellite countries, a fact kept secret in order to demonstrate the generosity of Moscow. By this method they aim at not only spreading Communism, but first of all Russian language, culture and Russian Communist imperialism. In the non-Communist countries, the loss goes on the account of the Soviet people. For instance, in France, Russian books are sold as cheap as in the Satellites. On the same terms one can buy any book, even the classics in Russian or originals, in a most artistic and solid binding. This attracts students and intellectuals in masses, from morning to late evening. The variety of the themes exceeds all that one can imagine.

The price the Russian reader pays for a book or a subscription for a current medical journal is well illustrated by the following examples which are 1960 subscriptions for the USSR (in old roubles):

1. Pediatrics (Pediatria) .... 42 Roubles
2. Clinical Medicine (Klinicheskaya Meditsina) .... 42 Roubles
3. Soviet Medicine (Sovetskaya Meditsina) .... 48 Roubles
4. Archives of Pathology .... 60 Roubles
5. Archives of Anatomy, Histology and Embryology .... 96 Roubles
6. Journal of the AM of USSR .... 72 Roubles
7. Bulletin of Experimental Biology and Medicine .... 96 Roubles
8. Journal of Surgery .... 72 Roubles

All of these Journals are monthly publications, the size of *The American Journal of Diseases of Children.*

The monthly salary of a Russian doctor is, on the average, seven to eight hundred roubles. You can then estimate what the one year subscription costs are in comparison to the salary. The reader can simultaneously estimate what portion of his monthly earnings an American doctor is paying for a year's subcription to a journal of any specialty. The same is true about books. To the Russian doctor they are not cheap. For instance, *T. P. Krasnobaev*, biography, size of an ordinary American textbook, 180 pages, 6 roubles; *The Teaching of Viruses*, by L. A. Zhilber, Moscow, 1956, format of American textbooks, 312 pages, 16.25 roubles! This same book is sold in Paris at a cost of 385 francs; that is one-fifth the cost in USSR at the dollar exchange rates in 1958 when the book was bought.

MEDICAL PERIODICALS

There is no better indication of the social, professional and scientific level of the doctor than the magnitude, kind and availability of medical literature. And of all literature, the periodicals containing the latest progress of medical science possess this significance in the greatest degree. There are 400,000 physicians in the USSR serving a population of 210,000,000. There are 42 periodicals directly linked with clinical medicine. All are the ordinary book size except *Soviet Medicine,* which is larger. Seventeen are monthly, one of which is a reference journal containing abstracts of current foreign medical literature. Of the others, 23 are bimonthly, one every 45 days and the other one quarterly. The clinical journals most widely circulated are:

1. *Klinicheskaya Meditsina,* monthly, publishing 40,000 copies.
2. *Sovetskaya Meditsina,* circulating 48,000 copies.
3. *Pediatria,* published in 44,000 copies.

All of these three journals have approximately the same number of pages, ranging from 90 to 150 each, ordinary book size. All started with a few thousand copies following World War II and gradually their circulation increased.

One must remember that these journals are widely spread throughout the entire Communist empire and beyond. This is not a voluntary, natural phenomenon, the result of the actual interest of the doctors abroad. This is a result of the servitude and subordination of the "satellites" and their Communist Parties to Moscow. Thousands of hospitals, institutions, libraries and doctors are, in most of the cases, involuntary or compulsory subscribers to those journals. So judgment about the precise spread of Soviet periodicals among the Russian physicians is impossible. We can, however, safely consider that about one-tenth of the copies go abroad. In such case, one copy remains for every ten to twenty Russian physicians. Interpreting this in its true meaning denotes nothing but scientific backwardness and more or less medical ignorance, poverty and apathy.

This becomes strikingly obvious when you take into consideration that 270,000 American doctors use over 300 clinical periodicals linked with clinical medicine; not to consider the publications of Great Britain as is the case with the *Lancet* and *British Medical Journal* which are widely circulated in this country; also Canadian, Australian and New Zealand periodicals. All of the American medical publications are private and they are received by the doctors on their own free choice. There are about 150,000 copies of the *J.A.M.A.* alone, issued weekly! The textual pages far exceed any of the Russian periodicals.

The character of the clinical articles in the journals is of a programmed nature, that is, most of the contents are relevant to mainly one problem elucidated from numerous aspects. Generally, articles prevail which deal with routine Soviet realities. At the same time, especially the academies and various institutes systematically sublist collective works, frequently of purely scientific character.

The stereotype of Soviet journals is characterized by the following features. The editorials are, as a rule, lengthy, with political, ideological or organizational subjects. The scientific articles are standardized to almost one short size. In the vast majority of cases they have summaries in Russian and another summary in a foreign language, in 75% of the cases, English.

Articles whose publication is rejected are given at the end of the journal in small type and in summary under "Annotations and Self-excerpts." More and more the sources are given, including the foreign ones. However, important journals like that of the *USSR Academy of Medical Sciences* and *Klinicheskaya Meditsina* have no summaries in a foreign language and not all of the articles are accompanied by a list of literary sources. The last portion of the journals is dedicated to various philosophical-scientific discussions and echoes on various subjects found in articles and books, Russian and foreign; excerpts of foreign literature are seldom given and in a very restricted degree because there is a special journal for this purpose. Finally, analyses and accounts are given of various Soviet and foreign conferences, congresses and meetings as well as obituaries in the language style already described.

What do the Soviet medical periodicals contain? There is, generally speaking, the routine dealing with the acute health realities of Communist society. Rarely can one encounter an original idea or article. Many times you can trace the origin of an article to Western sources, especially those of the U.S. On rare occasions it is done openly in order to have "verified" the reliability of "Western and Bourgeoise" scientists. Because medical periodicals are the truest expression of the level of medicine, in order to avoid waste of time, it is justifiable here to just quote the British doctor we have already mentioned above. Writes Dr. J. B. Horman: "What struck me about medical Russia was the Englishness of it all." By this, Dr. Horman means that there is nothing original; that it is copied. And as to that, the medicine most copied in the USSR is that of the U.S. As soon as U.S. publications are printed, they are carefully studied by special teams and institutions; first by the USSR Academy of Medicine, the planner of Soviet medical science, and thereafter the thematics and ideas are widely used, especially by the research workers and the academicians. Almost the only originality of Soviet medicine lies in Pavlov's teaching. Other originalities are servility and political madness to the extent of cowardice and crime.

There is no mention in the medical press of the social life of those in the medical profession because it simply does not exist. As to the professional-scientific life, the various conferences, symposiums, congresses and meetings relevant to the carrying on of the daily professional obligations and leadership of the Party in the health field, this is also scantily published except for events involving a large number of people. The daily meetings, in fact, are so many and take up so much of the doctor's time that their publication is neither advantageous nor possible.

TECHNICAL QUALITIES OF SOVIET MEDICAL LITERATURE

It would be unjust if we did not say a few words regarding the technical qualities of Soviet medical and other publications. Up to World War II there were only a few publications of non-medical nature which were sufficiently fitting the appellation of real, cultural attainments. The great majority of the scientific publications were unbelievably ugly and technically and materially inferior. With rare exceptions, the paper was the type resembling that used in the colonies for wrapping sweets sold on the streets.

This trend continued up to about 1947. (Publications were almost entirely discontinued during the war.)

Since that year, for the duration of about a year or so, the entire shape of all publications changed amazingly. Almost all (not the current publications) became outstanding and alluring! The so-called "Satellites" were flooded with virtually every publication of the Soviets, sold at numerous Russian bookstores in the capitals as well as in many other provincial cities.

How can we explain these rapid and fundamental changes? Intellectuals there attribute it to the German technicians, captives in the USSR. What depended on the latter became excellent, but what depended on the Russians themselves was, and is, almost unchanged to this very moment. For instance, up to a short time ago, the thing you had to look for first when you bought a Russian book was the page containing the errata. These pages were the regular accompaniment of every Soviet publication and contained only the "more important and noticed" errors. You have to look for hours to make the correction yourself and you are never sure that you are reading an authentic production. This has much improved recently.

A defect, (now much diminished) is the lack of a proper manner of giving the bibliography. In recent years there has been a tendency to follow the practice of the West and the U.S., but what is done is still insufficient. In the review of the various publications it is a frequent finding of the Russians to criticize themselves for this neglect and dishonesty. Summaries in a foreign language are not given even today in the *Journal of the Academy of Medical Sciences of USSR!* This is not accidental or due to lack of competent linguists. The omission leaves the coryphaei at liberty to sell Western science as their own. As to plates

and diagrams Soviet medical journals were poor, both
in quantity and quality but now they show progressive
improvement. Publications of translated foreign textbooks are rare. Only recently Fanconi-Wallgren's book
on Pediatrics was published in Russian.

EQUIPMENT AND FACILITIES

Here we wish to comment upon the conditions in
which the American and the Soviet doctor work.

In 1947, in Paris, on his return from the Second
International Congress of Pediatrics in New York and
a trip around the United States, Professor Robert
Debré, the oldest and of greatest renown among contemporary Europen pediatricians, told in extenso of
what he had heard at the Congress and seen in the
U.S. His first enthusiastic words were relevant to a
most striking impression of the American hospitals:
"their abundant equipment, equipment and equipment
and its very frequent replacement by newer, more modern equipment." True; I was struck by the same
reality. If one sees only the equipment on one of the
floors of Babies' and Children's Hospital at Western
Reserve University, Cleveland, Ohio, — if one only
sees the laboratories, the kind of incubators, even the
syringes and the needles, their number and the way
they are available for use, — if one sees what an amount
of material is used, for instance, of tape, or how many
meters of EKG paper or films are used for a patient,
— he will guess where some of the premises and the
roots lie of the unbelievable progress and achievements
of U.S. medicine.

Here is what a Soviet doctor, twice in two years a
visitor in the U.S., says:

"In them (the Americans) the drive to progress, toward everything new and advanced, is very great.

"Extremely great attention is paid in the U.S.A. to the question of creating laboratories at the medical, and especially the surgical wards; and to their equipment."

Here it what he says regarding what he saw in Houston, Texas:

"It should not go unnoticed that for every professor and assistant there are one or more secretaries. This undoubtedly leads to a more fruitful scientific work . . . In the surgical department of Professor DeBaky there are eighteen secretaries and one also administrative secretary — not a doctor." (F. G. Uglov, Impressions of a Visit to the U.S.A., *Klinicheskaya Meditsina*, March, 1962.)

What is the situation in the USSR, where the Russian doctor is confined to work? Dr. J. B. Horman (Great Britain) who visited the USSR in the summer of 1958 and was surely shown mainly propaganda objectives (hospitals) writes (*The Lancet*, 4-4-59):

"The routine laboratories (small) and apparatus for EEG, EKG and diagnostic radiology were there but somewhat old-fashioned. X-ray therapy seemed to be very limited. Clearly, government bounty had not extended to the hospitals."

The Vice President of the Academy of Medical Sciences of the USSR writes (*Herald AMS of USSR*, #9, 1961, p.27):

"Analyzing the reasons our research in the theoretical field is limited, it is necessary to point out that . . . contemporary science can progress only in conditions providing the needed, at times complex, equipment, reagents, etc. Lack of production in our country of such equipment sharply reflects upon the volume and the quality of the theoretical investigations. The equipment imported reaches the laboratories not earlier than two to three years after it is ordered."

Professor Walter Frajola (Ohio State University, Columbus, Ohio,) expressed the same opinion regarding the equipment, — recording "apparatuses" dating-like for example, from the time of Claude Bernard. He had seen it personally while in Moscow this last summer.

The truth is that the major technical equipment of Soviet hospitals is the X-ray apparatus, ultratherms and U.V.R. lamps. As a rule, most of the time at least one of them is out of order, sometimes for months, because of defective X-ray tubes, ultratherm mechanisms or U.V.R. bulbs. Frequently a cause of this is the carelessness of the personnel. Use of even one film is not considered justified for diagnostically "clear" patients; two films, or more than several centimeters of EKG paper carries the possibility of being considered a waste; if more material is "spoiled," what follows is remarks and warnings by the Party secretary or publicity in the newspapers.

It would take much time to cite the complaints of the Soviet doctors at the various local and all Soviet Union conferences regarding the lack of proper hospital laboratories to the extent that they are unable to cultivate diphtheria bacterium or to check up the sensitivity of the various pathogenic agents which are encountered on the media.

Following are excerpts from the discussions that have taken place with respect to the report of Professor N. N. Blohin (President of the Academy of Medical Sciences of USSR) and other reports before the Fifteenth Scientific Session of the General Assembly of the Academy of Medical Sciences of USSR. They illustrate the material, political and scientific status of the Soviet medicine. (*J. Acad. Med. Sciences of USSR*, #9, 1961).

"We should have in sufficient quantity and well purified, hormone preparations, reagents, etc.; equipping existing institutions and laboratories with the newest apparatus and well qualified cadres; create a plant producing endocrine preparation (E. A. Vassukova); testing sensitivity of infectious agents to antibiotics is of extreme importance but it meets difficulties because of the imperfection of the existing methods; pressing need for faster techniques (I. I. Rogozin); the question of Academy Equipment remains very unfortunate (V. V. Parin)."

This by itself, as read by our readers, is not at all horrible for the doctors. Nowhere is everything in perfect shape. But the control of the fulfillment of the tasks; reporting before the political organs of the institutions; the fear for delay of the fulfillment, and the necessity for one to lie in order to survive; the obligation to attend every meeting of ignorant and impudent Party organs; the predetermined fate by not being a member while those having Party membership represent the new privileged class; this all is mortally humiliating, offensive, and handicapping.

Scientific Organization of Soviet Medicine

The supreme administrative commander of Soviet medicine is the Ministry of Public Health. To it are subordinated in an administrative way all of the health institutions and health services in the Soviet Union. It carries down to the health bodies the various scientific problems in a practical manner. The Ministry of Public Health carries on this organizational and promotional work in close harmony with the Academy of Medical Sciences.

The Academy of Medical Sciences of the USSR

Any information regarding the activities of the Academy of Medical Sciences of USSR would be incomplete without a reference to the Institute of Experimental Medicine founded in 1888, in St. Petersbourg. There, almost from the beginning, Pavlov worked as its head. In 1932, it was reorganized and renamed ALL-UNION EXPERIMENTAL INSTITUTE OF MEDICINE. When World War II started, this institute, VIEM (from the initials of the Russian name) had a staff of five thousand scientific workers! In 1944, during World War II, the Institute was again renamed, the original name, Institute of Experimental Medicine, being retained by the Leningrad filial, and given autonomy, while the rest of the institution remained under the Academy. Today they number 280.

The Institute of Experimental Medicine alone was considered the main Institute and it was assigned to work in the field of Higher Nervous Activity, Biochemistry of Metabolism, Physiology of the Basic Function of the Human Organism and their nervous and humoral regulation.   Here Nikolai Krasnogorsky does research in the higher nervous activity in infants and children.

V. I. Lenin and the famous proletarian writer, M. Gorky, have played a great role in their tremendous contributions for the development of the Institute. From 1891 to 1940, the Institute published 9,000 scientific papers and monographs, 5,246 of them between 1930 and 1940.   Between 1955 and 1960, it has published 1659 works.

Today the Academy of Medical Sciences of the USSR is the almighty goddess of the entire Communist empire, including the so-called "satellite" nations. Among the medical sciences, it possesses as the most glittering and priceless diamonds of its crown, biology and Pavlov's physiology.   In its membership of several rankings it has hundreds of academicians who are the most outstanding men and women in both Science and the Party or in one or the other of them.   As a body it is something much larger and more complex than a ministry and its authority is incomparable to any other institution in the Soviet Union and is second only to the Central Committee of the Party.   Its staff, as a whole, numbers thousands upon thousands of scientific workers.

It is composed of divisions in all fields of medical sciences headed by secretaries and a group of members.   Every division has its scientific council.   The Academy as a whole has its Presidium presenting a kind of executive organ, and it also has its president and vice president.

The goals of the Academy are numbered from one to many tens upward.   Every problem has its group of "otgovornitsi," responsible members, of whom one is the "responsible-in-chief."

The amount of money the Academy consumes is hard for one to imagine. It gets from the Government anything it wants. If there are failures or retardations, they are due to bureaucracy, overstaffing, complexity, jealousy and confusion, all of which are typical of the Russian spirit and brilliantly depicted by the Russian classical masters, — Dostoevsky, Saltykov, Gogol, Chekhov, Zoshchenko and even the poet of the October Revolution, Mayakovsky who in disappointment committed suicide.

In fact, the Academy is a plant where, besides sound plans and goals being hammered out, great achievements are pledged or boasted of as though already attained. All this serves to cover the obvious inventive sterility, the barrenness in the purely scientific field as compared to the huge sums of money spent, the people involved in research and the humiliations suffered by the academicians. One has only to read the speech of the president of the Academy for the year of 1961 to be convinced of the correctness of our opinion. (Note: To avoid repetition, the reader will find excerpts of this speech elsewhere in this study.) It is really a sad evaluation.

However, the Academy is carrying on tremendous ideological, scientific research, training and practical organizational work. Following are a number of fragments of the labor complex which depict part of the image of the Academy, as well as some new steps toward improvement of its activities.

TABLE #1

THEMES	TOTAL	OF THEM		
		DOCTOR DIS.*	CANDI-DATES' DIS.*	MONO-GRAPHS
			* Dissertations	
1. Intestinal infections, dysentery mainly (Problem #16)	158	5	2	1
Of them:				
Dysentery	62	2	9	—
Typhoid fever and para-typhoids	44	2	2	—
Colibacilloses	26	—	1	—
Toxoinfections	26	1	—	1
2. Virus diseases, especially Grippe and Infections of the Upper Respiratory Tract (Problem #18)	167	6	10	1
Of them:				
Grippe	54	1	1	—
Infectious Hepatitis	55	4	3	—
3. Epidemic Poliomyelitis (Problem #19)	80	—	9	—
4. Hypertonic disease, arteriosclerosis and insufficiency of the coronaries (Problem #22)	262	12	42	5
Of them:				
Hypertonic Disease	103	4	14	4
5. Rheumatic fever and diseases of the joints (Problem #24)	391	16	60	4
6. Tuberculosis (Problem #27)	368	10	44	2
7. Malignancies (Problem #28)	545	28	63	12
8. Trauma, industrial, farm and life conditions, traumatism (Problem #29)	648	45	102	16
9. Angina, Chronic Tonsillitis (Problem #36)	338	19	38	7
10. Labor Hygiene and professional diseases (Problem #38)	234	11	—	4
TOTAL	3,561	166	400	57

Here is the program-plan of the Academy of Medical Sciences of the USSR relevant to ten most important themes for research carried on in the various institutions of health in the USSR during 1960 and conveyed by the Academy of Medical Sciences.

"The newly created Coordinative Commission at the AMS is destined to attract into cancer research not only medical men but also others from a number of adjacent institutions of the biological, chemical and physical profile." (President of the AMS of USSR, *Herald AMS of USSR*, #9, 1961.)

"In order that the material basis of the Academy may develop, the Construction-Montage-Repair Office in its system will be of significant importance; also, our Construction Bureau possesses a plant which is not large and the Academy is attempting to reorganize it; it is intended to construct new and perfected apparatus and instruments which are needed by the institutes of medical research.

"Taking into consideration the enlargement of the experimental work on the many important problems, and considering the necessity for a radical improvements in the raising of laboratory animals at the Academy, its presidium created a Special Laboratory for raising experimental animals . . ." (President AMS of USSR, N. N. Blohin, *Vestnik AMS of USSR*, #9, 1961.)

In the official scientific-organizational organ of the Academy of the Medical Sciences of USSR (Journal [Herald] of the Academy of Medical Sciences of

USSR, #7, 1961) we find such additional information as this regarding the activities of the Academy:

Problems of Organization and Planning of Science. Nearest Tasks of the Hygiene of Female Labor:

1. Meeting of the Scientific Council of the Institute of Obstetrics and Gynecology at the Academy of Medicine of USSR together with the Committee on this subject and the Peripheral Scientific Institutions.

2. Significance of Cytological Investigations in Medical Science.

Scientific Life of the Institutes. Department of Immunology and Oncology at the Institute of Epidemiology:

1. Basic Experimental works of the Department of Immunology and Oncology. (Enumerated are 57, of which 4 by Zilber have been published abroad.)

2. A Review of Doctors' Dissertations defended in 1957-1959 before the Scientific Council of the Division of Medico-Biological Sciences at the AMS of USSR. (These dissertations are not the same as for getting the doctor's degree in the West. They are by physicians of various ages who, after training through correspondence and scientific work, can aspire to a doctor's title.) Doctor of Medical Sciences is a title of great distinction, it is obtained by a very limited number of medics and bears a considerable increase of salary.

Conferences and Consultations. Scientific-Theoretical Conference at the AMS of USSR (Dedicated to the 90th Anniversay of V. I. Lenin's birth.) (The accounts of the conference occupy ten pages of small type.)

History of Medicine. The Scientific Heritage of I. I. Mechnikov. (Six pages of small type.)

Critics and Bibliography. Karabadini — A Therapeutic Book of the XV Century.

Invention. A simple apparatus has been invented by the Institute for "Inventing New Apparatus and Instruments" at the AMS, designed for puncturing and (1) obtaining material for biopsy, and (2) for determining the consistency of the liver with respect to discerning an ecchinococcus from cirrhosis or Ca. It has been found that the consistency of the ecchinococcus is hard like iron.

UNPRECEDENTED NUMBER OF MEDICAL CONFERENCES AND CONVENTIONS IN USSR

These present an attempt on the part of the leaders of Soviet medical science and its outreach into life, to compensate for the handicap to medical progress caused by the scanty information, the poverty of the Russian physician, and the negative effect of the Party upon the physician's creative will. It is safe to say that in the USSR more congresses and conferences occur on major scientific issues than in all the rest of the world. This has been going on for decades. For instance, in 1938 and 1939, a unique all-Union four day conference took place in Moscow. It dealt with the vitamins only. The transactions were published in detail in two volumes. The recommendations made at the time are still in effect for the Soviet physician! In 1955, the Eighth all-Union Conference of the Internists, which lasted four days, took place in Leningrad and was dedicated to the treatment with antibiotics. This last year the Fifteenth session of the Institute on Tuberculosis at the Academy of Medicine was held in Moscow and was devoted to the healing of tuberculosis. And so it goes, every fourth night all year long.

The conferences and congresses are often held at different localities. They are all-Union or regional and each time the coryphaei, specialists, present extensive reports, followed by discussions and the publication of the proceedings in sizeable volumes. The coryphaei attempt to bring the newest trends and achievements in medicine down to the isolated medical professionalists. The Academy carries on some of its Conferences in remote cities of the Union. Generally in relaying the information, the foreign sources are not mentioned. The following are a variety of examples:

Eighth All Soviet Union Conference
On the Use of Antibiotics in Internal Medicine
1955
(Works of Eighth All Soviet Union Conference of Internists, Medgis, 1956)

Professor E. M. Tareev, Moscow, internist, one of the most outstanding Soviet clinicians, author of a voluminous textbook on internal diseases, gave a report on "General Problems in the Use of Antibiotics in the Clinic." He used American sources and data without mentioning it. A. M. Sigal (Odessa,) thus commented on Tareev's report: "Many of the cases mentioned by Tareev regarding the side effects of antibiotics are widely described in the American literature."

Professor Z. V. Ermoleva, Moscow, one of the reporters, comments: "We have about eleven kinds of antibiotics, while abroad they have one hundred and sixty-three; at the present time in our Lazarev laboratory we have obtained a preparation with more prolonged action, — Bicillin."

L. I. Fogelson, Moscow, in his comments (page 212 of the same volume) says, "Since we do not have long acting preparations of penicillin, we have to introduce it I.M., no less than six, but better eight times in twenty-four hours!"

Other abstracts from the resolution of the conference: "Ask the Ministry of Public Health to improve scientific research with respect to finding new antibiotics, in particular, long acting preparations of wide spectrum type; speed up the production of the newest preparations, — Terramycin, Biomycin, Tetracyclin, etc.; improve the quality of the product with respect to the forms of the antibiotics; provide the necessary amounts of all antibiotics; supply us with the special apparatus for introduction of the antibiotics such as Aerosol; supply the clinics and large hospitals with bacteriological laboratories."

Scientific Session of the Institute of Pediatrics of the Soviet Academy of Medical Sciences, Together with Peripheral Institutes of Pediatrics, Moscow, 1959.

Participating in this session were 400 delegates, comprised of 40 professors, scientific workers from the scientific and medical institutions and medical schools, and 205 practical doctors from 44 cities in the various Soviet Republics.

Twenty-five reports were given on the problem of grippe; on pertussis, twenty reports; it was said that much was learned at this conference with respect to those two "wide-spread and grave infectious diseases of childhood." They are still lacking effective vaccine in sufficient amounts. A comparison of the originality of the themes and the opinions expressed at the conferences in USSR and in the U.S. indicates that the latter are far, very far, superior.

As an example it will suffice to only point out the last International Conference on Measles which was held in Bethesda, Maryland, November 7-9, 1961, or the one five years ago, The International Conference on Tuberculosis at the Jewish Hospital in Denver, Colorado, or any purely American conference or congress of any time in the last three decades. The standard is always of usually high scientific level; the seriousness, the honesty, and the modesty of American scientists and their concern to create science, not propaganda, have always been features of distinction. The clinico-pathological conferences of the Boston and Newark teams, the Friday mixed conferences or the Saturday conferences on the selection of the cases for open heart surgery at the Babies' and Children's Hospital at the Western Reserve University, Cleveland, Ohio, are events of which every American should feel proud.

There is another sign underscoring the freedom, the dignity and the democratism of this great country, the helping of one's self to coffee, tea and cookies during the time of the conferences; young or senior medical personalities all talk freely expressing their views. In USSR — the first thing one must have in mind is not to oppose a Party member or a chief. One has to think even whether to dare to say anything. For all is proper for and belongs to the coryphaei and the "big" men in the Party. As to the details we pointed out, they as a symbolization of freedom and equality are something unknown in the USSR.

PART II

BASIC SCIENCES

BASIC SCIENCES

BIOLOGY

Soviet biology pretends to present an "activated and higher" phase of Darwinism, that is, Michurinism. This term is from the name of I. V. Michurin, a semi-educated agronomist and selectionist who lived half of his lifetime before the October Revolution and half following it. It is noteworthy to mention that the real classical works on biology date from the epochs preceding the Revolution. Following it, one of the best of the very few exceptions is the work of V. P. Dobrohvalov which was produced in 1954. Though it is based on the routine Communist doctrine, it is one of the most honest, comprehensive and serious achievements in Soviet literature on biology and has nothing in common with Lysenkoist's charletanic and ignorant approaches.

Soviet biology differs from the West and the United States on several major points. 1. While Soviet biology accepts Darwin's teaching, it is desperately hostile with respect to the great naturalist regarding the existence of rivalry and strife within one and the same species and that this rivalry is a mechanism of natural selection. Led by dictatorial considerations, Communists deny the existence of this factor in man's species in order to insure obeisance to their despotic system. But a superficial look at Communist reality shows that they contradict themselves, for their order of Communism is a typical illustration of ruthless rivalry within the human species and even more, of persecution, oppression and destruction of one portion of the society by another, smaller portion. An unequivocal confirmation of this truth is the entire revolutionary theory of Lenin and the foremost classic of the October Revolution, M. Sholohov and his *Tihee Don* (Quiet Don) as well as the history of Russia and the Party itself. 2. The inheritance of Acquired Characters. Communist biologists maintain the thesis of the unity of the organism and environment. Recognizing that organisms have to change according to the requirements of the environment, they accept that those changes are inheritable.

U.S. biology maintains that environment determines changes, not through the inheritance of acquired characters, but by mutations of which only those survive that appear fitting the environment. Mutation is a deviation from the self-copying of living organisms in the process of their reproduction. This deviation is realized through changes in the very genetic substance transmissible from generation to generation. Some of the factors that are capable of inducing genetic changes are known to biology but most are not. However, today mutations are considered a phenomenon occurring at random and induced mutational factors appear insignificant in man's heredity. This is the most crucial problem in biology. Communists bring about Darwin's opinion which favors the inheritability of acquired characters. Unfortunately, as Western biologists now accept, Darwin's genius could not know more in his time, regarding these problems. The degree to which this paramount question is unclear to the advocates of the primary importance of the environment in the evolution of the species, is evidenced by the following citation from V. P. Dobrohvalov:

". . . In the process of species formation, the species' specificity of the organisms plays a great role, but what are the peculiarities of this role in the various species? What is the power of this species' specificity in the various periods of development of the organism? How is it manifested in respect to the conditions of existence of the species? To this and many other questions, there are no reliable investigations (that is, answers — author's note) up to this moment in our biological science." — V. P. Dobrohvalov: *Philosophical and Natural Science Premises of the Teaching of I. V. Michurin,* Moscow, 1954, p. 205.

Another fact increases the confusion in Communist biological ranks. In recent years it was widely accepted that the microbial resistance to the various antibiotics, after the latter were used for some time, is due to changes of the genetic information induced by the antibiotics.

Now it was established that the appearance of resistant types of microbes is due not to the direct influence of the antibiotics but to the presence of only a few microbes which, thanks to the mutations which are always occurring, pre-exist the introduction of a particular antibiotic. Other microbiologists say that antibiotics develop resistant types.

Of course change in the genetic information under the influence of various chemical and other factors remains a truth, but in man especially, the genetic information seems the least accessible to such effects

— accidental or planned, — and the changes the most ephemeral. The same darkness prevails in every corner of Communist biological "science."

The insusceptibility of men and especially youth to Communism proved the falsity of the boldest claim of Soviet biology from Sechenov to Michurin, that through environment, the younger the organism is, the easier it is changed. The reader can get a good opinion of the scientific standard of Soviet biologists by reading what one of the greatest contemporary biologists, Julian Huxley, says:

"All theories lumped together under the titles of orthogenesis and lamarkism are invalidated, including Lysenko's Michurinism which is now the officially approved theory of genetics and evolution in the USSR . . . indeed in the light of modern discoveries, they no longer deserve to be called scientific theories, but can be seen as speculations without due basis of reality, or old superstitions disguised in modern dress."

The above cited work of Huxley, as well as that of George Gaylord Simpson (American), *The Meaning of Evolution,* (p. 35, New American Library, New York,) have no counterpart in the USSR and behind the Iron Curtain. Meanwhile, the huge number of American Nobel Prize-winning scientists, — geneticists and other specialists, — justify quoting only this:

"Exciting things have been happening in genetics in the past few years, many of them directly or potentially relevant to the practice of medicine." (C. Frerer, Montreal, Canada, McGill University, 1958.)

Soviet biology, together with its mixture with Pavlov's teaching as interpreted by the most prominent biologists and physiologists (Pavlovists) sounds more like a philosophy than a science. Here is an example by the outstanding Pavlovist, P. F. Zdrodovsky, as published in the *J.A.M.S. of USSR*, #9, 1961.

"Earlier, based upon serological investigations, we found that in animals immunologically reactive, following over-stimulation, a refractory state takes place regularly. We interpreted this phenomenon as consistent with the dialectic regularity of the phenomena of excitation-inhibition as they were considered by N. E. Vvedensky.

"The immunogenesis is determined by non-specific neuro-humoral mechanisms controlling the biosynthesis of the proteins in general, which may be activated in particular by the antigen . . . this and other inferences dialectically unite the principle of the 'specific' and 'non-specific' and extend this principle also upon the action of the antigen."

The extent to which phantasies and violation of the bare facts of life were carried on by the prominent Pavlovist bio-physiologists is evidenced also by the following statements made by one of the most reliable biologist-virusologists of USSR today, L. A. Zilber, author of books and scientific papers. In his report before the division of Microbiology and Epidemiology at the Academy of Medical Sciences of USSR (*J.A.M.S. of USSR*, #10, 1961, p. 52) he writes:

"In the foundations of our contemporary understanding of the infection built up as a result of the classical works of Pasteur and Koch and the whole of the subsequent development of microbiology, three basic conditions lie:

1.   Infection (infectious process) presents per se the total biological processes originating from the interaction between the macro and the microorganism;

2.   Infectious process is always provoked by a live infection; and

3.   Motive (propelling) power of the infectious process all along, the infectious agent appears to be itself.

"The latter condition, in the thirties of our century, evoked active objections on the part of A. D. Speransky and I. V. Davidovsky (both foremost Pavlovists, note of G.T.,) who maintained that in the infectious process the microbe appears only as the 'historical point,' — that it starts the process but does not further participate in it, and the infectious process is moved ahead by self-motion.   However, the application of the antibiotics and chemo-therapeutic means definitely resolved the question.   It proved that the infectious process can be discontinued at any phase . . ."

We should add only that the conception of Speransky and Davidovsky was and is the official stand of the whole body of Soviet scientists, — biologists, microbiologists, infectionists.   For instance, all the writings and statements regarding Tuberculosis in the last fifteen to twenty years are deeply penetrated by this type of "science" of Nervism.   The same is true of the rest of the literature dealing with the relations of the infectious agent and the macroorganism.

The important thing is that mutations which Soviet

scientists considered idealistic creations, now are being accepted, but naturally again in the tendencious sense "that mutational changes are not random phenomena, not spontaneous ones, but are conditioned by causes from in and out of the organism."

The most remarkable phenomenon noticeable today in the field of biology is that Soviet biologists more and more frankly recognize the role of heredity in man's pathology. Before, it was anathema for anyone to dare to recognize the dominant role of constitution and heredity. For according to the dialectics, the whole matter depends upon environment. The apparent reversal is to the extent that Soviet biological scientists of today accept even the role of "heredity in Ca."

It seems that intensive research is going on in the field of restoring the vital functions of the organism hours after clinical death is induced. The latter is achieved by means of deep hypothermy which extends clinical death in dogs for two hours with subsequent complete recovery of all vital functions of the organism. Now they are attempting deeper hypothermy down to the degree of producing anabiosis. The experimenters (B. A. Negovsky, B. I. Soboleva, N. L. Gurvich, K. S. Kisseleva) are of the opinion that deep hypothermy opens great possibilities in the treatment of the terminal conditions, in heart surgery and in severe asphyxiation of the newborn. (*H.A.M.S. of USSR,* #10.) Another major field of great secret research is the tissue and organ transplantation.

But Soviet biology is still poor in research and achievements, even in the understanding of any crucial biological problem. This is evidenced by a glance only at the article of V. D. Timakov (Vice

President of the Academy of Medical Sciences of USSR) and A. G. Skavronskaya from the Institute of Epidemiology and Microbiology at the Academy of Medical Sciences of USSR. It is a leading article in #2 (Feb.), 1961, of the Academy's Journal. And in the bibliography only twelve Soviet sources are pointed out, while those of Western and mostly American origin amount to ninety. More than that, Russian sources cited are mostly summaries of what has been published abroad.

BIOCHEMISTRY

In the field of biochemistry more organized research is done in the USSR than in the whole Western world together. Biochemistry is a condition sine qua non for medical progress and the Russians have forgotten all their pretensions of dignity and greatness and in order to attain something they are in the role of parrots regarding their thematics of investigation. The most superficial acquaintance with their research reveals the extensive imitation especially of what is taking place in this field in the U.S. Many items of investigation, the terminology and the motivations you find months after they appear in the press of America and Western Europe.

Up to the present there is no one finding which has been recognized as completely original and especially one which has found beneficial application in the West. The most that they reach is half way. An example (rare) of this nature is the discovery of the Transaminase in the twenties by a Russian researcher. But he did not go farther. It needed the efforts in the U.S. of Cohen and co-workers in the early forties to exhaustively study this enzyme and establish its very important significance for the clinics.

That the above evaluation is correct is obvious from the following facts. Professor P. Brauner (Romanian, Bucharest) published an article in the leading Soviet Clinical Journal, *Klinicheskaya Meditsina*, #7, 1961, entitled "On the Enzymogram in Chronic Hepatitis and Liver Cirrhosis." After enumerating six such enzymes and commenting, he points out the thirty sources of reference and among them not one Russian, though the least conventional courtesy requires some sort of tribute to the host's pride.

Still more indicative are the following admissions. During the discussions at the Medico-Biological Division at the Academy of Medical Sciences of USSR which took place last summer it was said:

1. By Professor Dr. C. B. Anichkov, Director of the Department of Pharmacology at the Institute of Experimental Medicine of USSR: "Why is there with us, honestly speaking, a lagging behind that which is achieved abroad? The whole matter relates to the lagging of our chemistry."

2. By Professor C. Y. Arbusov: ". . . The pharmacology of our fatherland is considerably lagging."

3. By Professor L. L. Vassilev: "It was said, 'Our pharmacologists are lagging in comparison with those abroad . . .' I admit it is the neglectful attitude toward the physiological methods of investigation."

N. N. Blohin, the present President of the Academy of Medical Sciences of USSR, said the following with respect to the situation of the basic medical sciences and medicine itself in the Soviet Union and in the West:

"In the development of Soviet medical science and in the work of the Academy of the Medical Sciences of USSR serious defects exist as a result of which the tempo and scope of scientific investigation no longer meet the increased needs of protection of health and our country's economy, and in some important fields, there is a lagging of our fatherland's medicine behind what is found abroad. This especially relates to the fundamental theoretical research in virusology, cytology, genetics, biochemistry and immunology, all of which unveil new perspectives of prophylactics and treatment." (Leading article dedicated to the forthcoming XXII Party Congress, published in the official organ of the Academy, *Vestnik [Herald] of the Academy of Medical Sciences of USSR*, #9, 1961.)

Where the Soviets are in biochemistry is obvious from the proceedings of the Fifth International Congress of Biochemistry which took place in Moscow (August 10, 1961). At this Congress 1900 reports were read and 1596 discussions were carried on. Two plenums were held on two themes, the first reported by the U.S. representative (B. E. Green,) on the subject of "The Structure of the Subcell Particles."

In the account about the work of the Congress given by the doctor of biological sciences, E. A. Govorovich (Moscow,) published in the December issue of *Klinicheskaya Meditsina* (1961) there is no information regarding any remarkable report done by the Soviet delegates whose number has been the largest.

Naturally pharmacology, biochemistry, chemistry and clinics are linked and are mutually dependent one to another. It means that in all these fields the Soviets are lagging and this is obvious from the facts of this paper.

PHYSIOLOGY AND PAVLOV'S TEACHING

Physiology is inseparable from medicine, says Pavlov, and simultaneously he, by means of his physiological teaching, gave the strongest substantiation of the idea of Nervism which was first initiated by Botkin. The essence of this idea of Nervism, which encompasses Soviet medicine from beginning to end, is this. Organism is a unity and this unity is realized, directed and controlled by the nervous system. "All of the organism's processes," says K. M. Bikov, the greatest living Pavlovist, "are subordinated to the nervous organization in the normal as well as in the disturbed course of vital functions. There is no branch in medicine where the first role does not belong to the Pavlovian concept of the course of organism's functions. American *psychosomatic medicine* is a weak and monstrous echo of the Russian idea of Nervism. Psychosomatic medicine, especially in the United States, where the monopolistic capital most impudently shows expansionistic tendencies, has for grounds the concept that the cause of neuroses is rooted in the lower instincts of people and in the civilization infringing upon these instincts. But at the same time those people and their civilization are considered out of the class struggle of the Bourgeoise society." In the same bitter language Freudism is negated, as encouraged by "the reactionary circles, mainly in Great Britain and the United

States, a dogma and practice which was outmoded a long time ago as anti-scientific."

Fundamental recognition is given by all Pavlovists to Pavlov's concept regarding the long lasting focuses of excitation in the brain cortex. These focuses can maintain pathological processes in the organism for an indefinite time and independently of the causative agent and the treatment. This phenomenon is known as the "Dominant of Ukhtomsky." The latter has the capacity to draw to its realm and thrive upon any new excitation which takes place in the cortex though unrelated to the basic pathological process from which the Dominant originated. It became convenient for the Soviet Pavlovists to most easily find such development in the chronic diseases. Tuberculosis thus became the territory where this philosophy appeared most conspicuous. In this respect an example was for years widely commented upon and pointed out, — the case described by M. V. Trius, a lady phthisiologist. The case concerned a man who for many years had had active pulmonary tuberculosis and had died because of it. But his believed specific flora, that is BK, had proved absolutely non-pathogenic! This unveiled "another" characteristic of the relation: macro-microorganism, — the microorganism being only the trigger for the pathological process whose further course is independent, going on on its own. This concept, which we mentioned previously, is, according to the Pavlovists, one of the paramount proofs of the role of the nervous system.

Unfortunately this theory is in basic opposition to the rest of the concepts of Pavlovism, or Nervism, as they alternately name it. According to Nervism, the nervous system is maintaining the equilibrium between the organism and the environment from which the former is "an inseparable part;" the nervous system is the main adjusting factor. In other words, the nervous system masters the survival, in health and in disease.

But how does it happen that pathological processes which are inconsistent with the maintenance of life develop in the organism? Well, the answer is easy for the Pavlovists. They say the nervous system is the organizer of the defensive processes, not of those giving up life. They say so presumably because the nervous system can only be the promoter and protector of life . . . We should not forget that the analogue of such a nervous system is the Communist Party in human society. Such is the hidden role that Communists ascribe to themselves.

It is up to the reader to weigh the value of this Soviet science, as well as to make his own conclusions regarding the theory that the bacterial agent is only the trigger factor of the pathological process. How can any pathological infectious process be stopped by antibiotics at any moment if there is not a bacterial agent which maintains it?

"There is no limit to the fluctuations and changes that can be induced in the higher nervous activity of man," says Pavlov, "if there are available for that, favorable conditions. Anything can be attained in the proper circumstances," he claims again regarding the nervous processes in man. His most outstanding adherent, academician Bikov, wonders how it is possible that such negligible things as the beat of the metronome or the sound of the bell are capable of causing such grave disorders in the experimental dog. Why not? All of Pavlov's experiments in connection with the neuroses were carried out in abnormal conditions for the animal. It ultimately had a nervous breakdown or died. Had it been free it never would have had the disorder, as wild animals never have them. In following its instinct of freedom, the animal ignores the strongest of other instincts, that of survival. Says Pavlov, "The fundamental nervous reactions, both in man and animals, are inborn in the form of reflexes and all of the remaining nervous activity of the organism is based on these reflexes." And in a highly demonstrative language, he draws the attention of scientists and surely of politicians, sociologists and statesmen, that "there does exist an unnoticed inborn reflex (instinct) which is of greater power and significance than any other. It is the freedom reflex." He writes further:

"As we know, in some animals the freedom reflex is so strong that when placed in captivity, they reject food, pine away and die . . . it is obvious that the freedom reflex is one of the most important reflexes, or to use a more general term, reactions, of any living being."

These truths are of vital theoretical, scientific, ethical and practical meaning. How do the Russian Pavlovists, physiologists, manage to transplant them on the biosocial field, in the society and the individual? How do they explain to themselves the continuous flow of people from behind the Iron Curtain to the West? The Hungarian Resurrection and that of the Tibetans? Absolutely unconcerned are those scientists about the obligation to give a reasonable answer. This shows only one thing, — that the so-called disciples of Pavlov are practicing a kind of metaphysical "physiology." Or to repeat the illustrative, purely Russian, Tolstoyan language, Soviet scientists, physiologists, Pavlovists, read and apply physiology and Pavlov's teachings as the Devil reads and applies the holy Gospel. However, we should have a little more mercy for them; they reach that far because they are paid to go so far and no farther. In fact, they serve well their bosses, pouring flames against the Western world, especially the U.S. "where monopolistic capital most impudently shows expansionist tendencies." (Academician K. M. Bikov.)

Soviet Pavlovist physiologists claim that they have another great merit in the establishment of the "natural regularities of equality" in human society. This they achieve through their concept of labor, physical and mental. As all of man's actions are carried on by the nervous system, and as all man does, according to Pavlov, is a reflex, therefore there is no other difference between physical and mental labor except one of degree. So the workers have to be happy and consider themselves mental laborers with the miserable pay they get from the same Government which is so generous in dealing with the real intellectuals who receive many privileges and very high salaries, and not one but several at the same time. As to the equality, it is shown on the pages of this short paper as well as in the book, *The New Class* by M. Jilas.

Scientists, especially doctors and academicians, are considered all over the world as the most democratic people; such, particularly, should be those who preach the highly noble, humanistic teaching of Pavlov. It is not that sort of people that we find the high ranking Russian doctors to be.

It was in 1945 that the Soviet army invaded Bulgaria and settled in many barracks, institutions and localities. The Tuberculosis Hospital at the capital of Sofia was occupied also and served the Soviet army. Some of the personnel, including some doctors, were Bulgarian, attached to serve the "brothers" from the USSR. One of these doctors was a lady, Dr. Y., who was known as an ardent pro-Communist, if not actually a Communist. "I am greatly disappointed and disgusted," she told me one day. "We," she went on, "take our meals at the hospital because of our bad supply and the great privileges the USSR army has. We were doing that in one room which was supposedly serving all of us and all of the Russians as well. But I was puzzled because only the lower ranks of Russian officers were dining with us. I expressed curiosity, asking a lieutenant doctor to explain to me the absence of the 'big' officers and doctors. I was shocked by this doctor's answer.

" 'We are categorized in several groups,' he said. 'The chief doctor, a colonel, does not communicate with any of us in the lower ranks. He eats alone. The ranks up to major communicate and eat together but in a separate room, while we, the lowest ranking officers, are here with you.'

" 'How is it possible?' I objected; 'Such inequality!'

" 'Do not wonder and protest,' the young doctor said. 'If I dare say anything directly to the big doctor I would get into the greatest of trouble. This is forbidden'."

It is logical to ask, what are the achievements of Pavlovists in the various fields of medicine. The answer could be a very simple one, — it is a complete failure. The proof? Here it is. The treatment of peptic ulcer through deep sleep in the course of three to four weeks; the suppressing of hypertensive disease (hypertension) by means of changing environment and conditioned reflexes; tissue therapy which admittedly should influence the organism's nervous system and thus be curative in every illness; fortifying the nervous system by biogenic stimulators and thus turning to the good the course of infectious diseases, of the malignancies, etc., etc., all proved a complete failure.

It is noteworthy that in recent years, in this late Khrushchev era, much less good is said of Pavlovism and its absolute domination of Soviet medico-biological thinking is less recognized. This is evidenced by the scant and reserved attention that Pavlov and the achievements of his disciples received in the evaluation on the occasion of the twenty-second Party Congress. Following are the appraisals of the President of the Academy of Medical Sciences of USSR, N. N. Blohin, as we find them in the *Herald of the Academy of Medical Sciences of USSR*, #9, 1961, p. 17.

1. "It is necessary to mention that our physiologists (all are Pavlovists, — author's note,) who, several years ago, were making great pledges with respect to further creative development of the scientific heritage of our great I. P. Pavlov, in recent years principally have made little new investigation of the higher nervous activity. In the report of the president of the 'Problems Commission,' the member-correspondent of the Academy of Medical Sciences of USSR, D. A. Birukov, the achievements announced are not of very great significance. For instance, it is said that through the aid of special methods there had been established weakness and quick exhaustion of the processes of excitation and inhibition in oligophrenics, or that in little children conditioned reflexes to

speech as a stimulator are formed more slowly than to the direct stimulators, while in adults the reverse is true. As carriers of this latter investigation, two institutes are pointed out, — the Institute of Physiology at the Academy of Medical Sciences of USSR and the Institute of Pediatrics at the Academy of Medical Sciences of USSR.

"We very often are inclined to attribute all of our failures to the insufficient equipment of institutes and laboratories. However, many of the defects in the working out of the most important problems are not linked with it. On the contrary, many of the institutions are not at all inadequately equipped and they have favorable conditions for a considerable improvement of their work." These are bitter though courteous criticisms that are directed at the Pavlovists.

2.   In the field of Pediatrics the most outstanding researcher-scientist is N. Krasnogorsky (see also the chapter on Pediatrics). He works at Leningrad and is the Director of the Pediatric Institute at the Academy of Medicine of USSR. His name was completely absent from the vast number of reports, commentators and scientists of merit on the occasion of the XXII Party Congress. This fact, by itself, speaks more than anything with respect to the sad condition in which the Pavlovists have placed themselves.

3.   A resolution of the Consultation on the Question of the Higher Nervous Activity of Man was taken December 26, 1960. In this consultation in Moscow there were physiologists, psychologists, scientists, psychiatrists, pediatricians and neuro-

pathologists. Following the reading of a number of reports, and discussions, the Consultation found:

I. That in the studies on the problems of the higher nervous activity of man, a series of achievements have been attained.

II. That there are defects and difficulties in the studies of the higher nervous activity of man. The consultation further complained because of the small number of physiological, psychological and clinical institutes carrying on the research in this field. Further, the consultation points out that "Scientific research is not coordinated sufficiently; it meets the needs of practice but little, and is carried on without sufficient adherence to the contemporary methodology." (*Journal of Neuropathology and Psychiatry honoring S. S. Korsakov,* #5, 1961.) This all reveals a backwardness and futility in USSR along the lines of creative research and achievement in the field of the higher nervous activity of man.

The sad and shameful excesses in the USSR in every field of society were absolutely copied in the so-called "Satellite" nations of which my country of Bulgaria holds the second place in the camp of the Communist world. Anything that appears in those small countries whose tyrant is Moscow, is an echo only of what is going on in the USSR. So the story of Orbelli and colleagues we mentioned in the beginning of this paper has an analogue in Bulgaria which is worthy of being described. It was in 1950, shortly after the combined session of the USSR Academy of Sciences and USSR Academy of Medical Science was held in Moscow. It was dedicated to the development and the ingraining of Pavlov's teaching of Nervism into the rest of the Medico-Biological fields.

The Bulgarian delegation which represented our country, on its return from the USSR, held a special session of all scientists and professionals linked in one way or another with physiology, medicine and the biological sciences. Everybody was speaking and bowing to "Pavlov." Vast "experimentation and application" of Pavlov's teaching were started. Not a long time later conferences were held at which reports were read relevant to the successes achieved. One of these reports dealt with the treatment of peptic ulcer with stomach juice of healthy persons induced into the stomachs of the victims of peptic ulcer! The grounds? Pavlov's conceptions regarding the immunological properties of the saliva and stomach secretion. The results? Good. The fate of the discovery? Forgotten. The authors of the research and the achievements? Dirty opportunists who were doing similar research under the Nazi domination.

At one time, 1921-26, there was a professor at the State University of Sofia by the name of Vassilii Zavialov. He was a Russian and taught normal physiology. He and his family were escapees from the October Revolution. He was one of the most brilliant intellects one could ever meet. Two decades later, in the Communist era, his son, Vsevolod Zavialov, also became a professor in physiology at the second University of Plovdiv, Southern Bulgaria. He was an even more brilliant and broadly gifted man than his father was. Observing the humiliating worship of Pavlov he was so uncautious as to say before one of his colleagues, "When will this Pavlovmania ever end?" The "kind colleague," a spy and a mean Communist, immediately reported to the Rector of the University, Dr. Kristanov, a Bulgarian trained in Russia. In three days the faculty and the university corps of professors were summoned and "unanimously" voted the expulsion of the brilliant man from the university.

There is moderation now in the realms of Pavlovism, in fact, pseudo-Pavlovism. It is already noticeable and will grow as Stalinism fades away. What was wrong with Pavlovism? It was not Pavlov that was wrong but the Pavlovists. For in their servitude to the Party and their dishonesty they tried to knock out from the domain of physiology every sound understanding of man and identify Pavlov's teaching regarding the mechanisms of psychic activity with the psychic activity itself. Thus they provided the Party with a method and a "science" through which the changing of man and the ingraining of Communism was an easy task.

On the questions, what are the essentials of Pavlov's teaching, and what are the impacts in the clinics? The answer is confined to the following:

1. It scientifically, abundantly and complexly substantiated the idea of Descartes that nervous reactions are reflexes;

2. That all nervous reactions are carried on by means of conditioned and unconditioned reflexes;

3. That in favorable conditions such reactions can be produced as desired;

4. That besides the reflexes another element in nervous activity is the existence of two fundamental nervous processes — excitation and inhibition.

In view of these mechanisms the teaching illuminates the roads of scientific ethics and soundest pedagogy, physiology and prophylaxy.

While this was happening among the Soviet Pavlovists regarding physiology, in the U.S. physiological science was following the paths of Claude Bernard and thus clearing the way towards obtaining the information that underlies the epochal successes of U.S. medicine.

Pathological Anatomy

Pathological anatomy holds a place of highest esteem in medicine. Soviet pathological anatomy has its masters, among whom, of particular merit and the most outstanding are V.G. Shtefko and A. Abrikossov, the latter being the author of a very popular two-volume textbook of the same discipline written in a classical manner and based on material of his own.

Soviet pathological anatomy has one great virtue and that is the existence of a separate Pediatric Pathologoanatomical school headed by two notable pathologists, V. T. Talalaev and M. A. Skvortsov, and hundreds of other pathologists, most of them being their disciples. This achievement appears to be of great significance in view of the extraordinary importance of the pathology of infancy and childhood in general pathology and medicine as well.

In pediatric pathological anatomy the most outstanding pathologist is A. I. Strukov. He has published 130 papers and two books on pediatric pathologoanatomy. He was a disciple of Professor A. Abrikossov. Strukov has highly specialized in the field of the pathological anatomy of tuberculosis.

Soviet pathologoanatomists have done and are doing a colossal amount of work. Unfortunately apart from the routine, "black" job, they have little to be proud of.

This, however, does not prevent them from pretending priority in invention or originality, on the one hand, or from "checking up" the reliability and honesty of what is achieved abroad, on the other hand. Their pretension to have discovered what is unquestionably the discovery of the West is a result either of ignorance or of dishonesty and fear of the Party which demands results and a pay-off for the esteem it holds for science and scientists. Some role in this manner of participation in the world scientific scene may originate from consideration of national pride which is a powerful drive of every Russian.

In reviewing the merits of the Soviet pediatric anatomo-pathological school, Professor A. B. Volovik (*Forty Years of Achievements in the Field of Combat Against Rheumatism in Children,* Pediatria #12, 1957,) attributes it to these findings:

1. Rheumatic granulamotosis may remain latent and undetected by the clinician.

2. The severity of cardiac damage is determined by the non-specific exuditive-infiltrative changes.

3. Heart failure of varying degrees may ensue before myocardial sclerosis has taken place.

4. Mitral stenosis with insufficiency is much rarer in children than in adults.

5. Primary carditis and chorea are much more frequent in children than the arthritic form of rheumatic fever.

6. The heart might not be involved in the first attack, but by the second.

7. In children involvement of the joints plays a lesser role, but the vascular system is often involved, especially in rheumatic coronaritis.

If not naivity, is this not all an impudence? For all this has been known in the West for no less than 40-50 years.

However, Soviet pathologists have several achievements which impress the Western student and are worthy of being pointed out. First, there are the changes of the nervous system caused by the various toxic factors. The following functional disturbances do not correspond to the degree of pathologoanatomical damage. The knowledge of this allows the clinics to have a more correct account of the course of the various illnesses. These changes in the peripheric nervous system were conspicuously revealed in tuberculosis. Another finding of interest was the allergy as a local phenomenon. This idea of "local allergy" as a pathogenic factor in tuberculosis was formulated first by Ravich-Shterbo, outstanding phthisiologist who died ten years ago and whose remarkable book on pulmonary tuberculosis evoked more discussions in the Soviet Union than any other. The changes in the nervous system with the sequelae anticipated on the basis of Nervism reveal the mechanism of obscure pleurisies on the side where the greatest tuberculous lesions are located and as it was said, with changes in the peripheral nervous system not running parallel to the same lesions.

Much of this is debatable as in the live patient it is impossible to always make verification; and even if it is true, we do not have specific means to combat the functional changes of the nervous system. Much of this discussion and pretension seems to be more speculation than practical science. We have mentioned it, however, because it presents some original approach.

Another claim of priority by the Soviet pathologoanatomists is that they were the first to describe that in the primary tuberculosis infection, the lymph nodes caseificate as a whole, while in the post primary phase they caseificate at their "poles," with only part of the cortex.

Very interesting findings were established by Soviet neuropathologists in the field of brain development in man and the effect of various deleterious factors on it. The essence of the findings is confined to the role of the function of the nervous system of the fetus; that in the latter the vestibular apparatus first starts functioning through the stimulation of the skin receptors. This stimulation ultimately enhances the development of the cortical analyzer centers and the status of one of these analyzers affects the state of the other. They support this claim by means of following up the effect of asphyxia of the fetus intra- and extrauterinam, the effects of the regime of the pregnant woman, of some drugs, etc. When function is discontinued, brain development is impaired.

The one field in which Russian pathologists can claim contributions, but again with lack of originality, is the central nervous system. Here they have two achievements: (1) It is their *Atlas of the Cytoarchitectonics of the Cortex of the Main Brain of Man,* which appeared in 1955. As it is the second of its kind in the world, the first atlas being to the credit of K. von Economo, 1925, much less detailed, and old, the achievement of Soviet neuropathologists is of great significance. (2) The works of U. G. Shevchenko dedicated to the individual and group variations of the cortex of the main brain of contemporary man. His work appeared in 1956 and comprises the pathological findings in the lower parietal region of 52 brain hemispheres: Russians-41, Jews-6, French-2, Germans-1, Chinese-4 brain halves, Buriates-1, whose two hemispheres have been investigated. The conclusion of the author is: "There is no scientific proof that the brain of some tribes or races of contemporary humanity are the intermediate link between the brain of the monkey and the brain of the white races." Therefore, he maintains, *there are no higher and lower races and denounces racism of any sort.*

In one of the recent Soviet medical journals we found the description of a fatal case in which the opinion of the pathologoanatomists seems highly justified. For this reason we take the liberty of relating it briefly.

A woman patient had been continuously vomiting but clinical investigations and treatment had not helped in the least. The woman died and the pathologists found only two pathological changes, — scars on the right side of the neck (scrophulosis) and in the right basis of the lung an infiltration. These findings and the arrythmic pulse and rate of 40 had led the pathologists to the conclusion that the vagal nerve had been pressed by the two mentioned pathological formations and the incurable vomiting caused the fatal outcome.

Meanwhile, great attainments were registered in the West in recent years in the field of pediatric pathologoanatomy. These achievements, either with their originality or elaboration, belong, for the most part, to U.S. pathologists.

Pediatric pathology does not have the status of a formal subspecialty in the U.S. Rather, it is a group of general pathologists with pediatric interests working in or near the larger centers of pediatric practice. The first such pathologists in this country were Maude Abbott, whose fundamental work in the pathology of congenital heart disease is well known; Dorothy Anderson and Sidney Farber. Farber's department was established in Boston in the 1930's and has been the most important center for the training of pediatric pathologists in the country. There are a number of pediatric anatomopathologists, one who is highly promising being Dr. Robert Bolande, on the staff of Western Reserve University.

The most important books used in this area are: E. L. Potter, *Pathology of the Fetus and Newborn,* J. E. Morrison, *Fetal and Neonatal Pathology,* and R. A. Willis, *The Borderland Between Pathology and Embryology.* Two years ago there appeared the first complete pediatric anatomopathology by D. Stowens, 676 pages, large format.

In American pediatrics, pathology has been of monumental importance in the modern understanding of congenital heart disease. The work of Maude Abbott has been mentioned in this regard. The work of Anderson and Farber has been very important in developing our understanding of the fibrocystic disease of the pancreas. In a similar manner is the truth of the maple syrup urine disease, collagen diseases, toxoplasmosis, hyaline membrane disease, etc.

In Madrid at the IV International Congress of Clinical Pathology (June 13-17, 1960,) Soviet clinicians did not present one single report, though 200 such reports were read on Immunology, Ferments in Laboratory Diagnostics, Tissue Cultures in Bacteriological, Virusological and Parasitological Diagnostics,

Hormones and their Application in Diagnostics, Differential Diagnosis of Jaundices, and Organ Biopsy in Clinical Diagnostics.

The Soviet Union was represented by a five member delegation, headed by member correspondent of the AMS of the USSR, Professor I. A. Kassirsky. He it is who gives the account of the work of the Congress and says this with respect to the activity of his delegation at the Congress:

"I A. Kassirsky came up into the discussions with extensive analysis of the American data and in general the data found in the medical literature and also some of the experience of Soviet authors in the field of transplantation of bone marrow. Having subjected to a review the works of the American authors (in which the tendency was felt of very daring clinical experiments in the radiation of patients) he pointed out that . . ." (*Journal of the AMS of USSR*, #11, 1960, pp. 76-81.)

While the Soviet scientists were "subjecting to extensive analysis" the works of the American and other delegations, reports were read by delegations of such small nations as Italy, Spain, Belgium and Switzerland. The U.S. delegation made six reports, — more than any other delegation.

PART III

CLINICAL SCIENCES

CLINICAL SCIENCES

HEMATOLOGY

In the post-war epoch, thanks to the contributions of American clinicians and investigators, hematology made tremendous advance, especially in the realm of the pediatric age group.

Conversely, Soviet hematology is the poorest in contributions of any magnitude and clinical recognition abroad. Leaders in post revolution general hematology are M. I. Arinkin and, of a later date, N. N. Bobrov, who mostly studied the white hemogram of the tuberculosis patient, basing his knowledge upon clinical and experimental cases. Particularly pretentious was his opinion regarding the hemograms of tuberculous organism with various forms and phases of the infection. His findings are confined mainly to the relation of the four main types of white blood corpuscles, — an elevation of the monocytes being indicative of an active or reactivated tuberculous process. Another prominent hematologist is I. A. Kassirsky.

It is claimed by Professor Toor, one of the outstanding Soviet pediatricians and academicians, that "Bobrov and Soviet pediatricians have, contrary to previous concepts, established first in the world that in primary tuberculosis the number of neutrophils can be well over 10,000." Alas, everybody knows that this is not Soviet merit, — that it is an old, old story of which only the ignorant now boast.

In the middle twenties, Mikhailov, a phthisiologist, described a blood test destined to reveal by "titration" whether a tuberculous patient has active or inactive tuberculous infection.   In case of active infection, the eosinophils should suffer the so-called "eosinophilic shock."   Then in the peripheral blood they diminish 30% or more following the introduction of 0.10 cc. old tuberculin of the sixth dilution. The blood is rechecked thirty minutes later.   Other Russian phthisiologists claim that "this test has met with great approval abroad."   As it would appear most useful in the pediatric age, it is worthy to point out that it is not even mentioned in any of the Western classical textbooks of pediatrics, — Debré's, Fanconi-Wallgren's and Waldo-Nelson's last, seventh, edition of 1959.

Another author, Panchenko, invented a micro method of sedimentation of red blood corpuscles.   It is used in children and infants by means of a drop of blood only.   Otherwise it follows very nearly the figures of Westerngren. Micromethods have been also practiced in the West long before Panchenko in USSR. As to the use of correction and prerequisites of an ideal performance, there is nothing of that sort in the Soviet method.

Russians also are proud that they have found a bottomless well of human blood, and thus have solved the crucial problem of blood supply in peace time and in emergencies of any kind.   This is the blood of the dead patient corpses, withdrawn within six hours after death.   Blood is considered by the Russian teaching of Nervism the mightiest "biogenic factor" or stimulator of human organism.   Years ago it was widely used intramuscularly in a great number of clinical entities. Recently fractioned transfusions are favored more than in any other country. One does not find, in their current medical literature, any reservation toward this method which is questioned in the West because of a number of untoward effects, including the danger of infectious hepatitis, syphilis, mistakes, etc.

However, the classification of the anemias, blood discrasias, infectious mononucleosis, sickle cell anemia, gamma globulin with its adjacent abnormalities and its effect against some infections and ending with Rh factor, auto-agglutinnic anemias, leukemias, exchange transfusions and Coomb's and Paul Bunnell-Barrett tests, Russian hematologists have nothing in common with. All these and numerous other distinctions above all belong to American medicine.

I. I. Balashova described the first case of Congenital Agammaglobulinemia in the USSR (*Pediatria* #10, 1958,) and she writes, "There is not one other communication on this intriguing and important item which was first discovered in the U.S. by Bruton O. C. in 1952."

In a review of *Forty Years' Achievements of Soviet Pediatrics*, Professor A. F. Toor comments on hematology in only three lines, saying that major problems are still unsolved. Nothing is said about the problems the Soviet hematology has resolved. In the review of the achievements of Soviet medicine since the XX Congress (1956) by the president and vice president of the Academy of Medical Science of USSR, there is not one word for any merits in hematology. (*Herald of the AMS of USSR*, #9, 1961.)

In the important field of leukemias there is not one contribution of significance. It is recognized that "works in the USSR dedicated to bone marrow blood formation, are comparatively few." This is from an article by G. S. Moukhamesianova, on the staff of the Older Children's Institute of Pediatrics at the Academy of Medical Science of the USSR, second in the row of the Journal (*Pediatria*, #6, 1957.) The early laboratory diagnosis is built on the WBC and differential of the peripheral blood and, "if necessitated," of the bone marrow. Nothing is said about the reticolocytes, blood chemistries and cerebrospinal fluid, its cell contents and the X-ray findings. This methodology, compared with the American, looks like the naivity and the incompetence of the doctors thirty years ago.

According to dialectic philosophy and O. B. Lepeshinskaya — that life originates from living matter, not only from cells as Wirchow maintained in his famous *Omnis cellula e cellula,* and that this process does continuously occur, "K. A. Lavrov of the Rostov Institute of Medicine (medical school) established the great plasticity of tissues and the possibility of transforming living muscular fiber substance into red blood corpuscles." This is considered as a proof substantiating the irregular and changing blood picture of the leukemias. Lepeshinskaya's thesis also is that as life has generated billions of years ago, so today it generates out of the living matter.

E. V. Sergeeva (1958) investigated the dynamics of phagocytosis in diphtheria, measles, dysentery, typhus fever, infectious hepatitis, pertussis and in a number of other infections. Her findings show that "phagocytosis increases in every infection and decreases when infections are secondary complications or in the allergic phase." It is also accepted by them that grown children have better phagocytic activity than younger; antibiotics do not decrease phagocytosis while biogenic stimulators do!

O. M. Lago found that in prolonged grave intoxications and acute toxicoses, in the first place, the monocytic reactivity of the macroorganism is inhibited while the neutrophilic remains often quite active. Inhibition of only the monocytic reactivity paralleled by active neutrophilic is not an unfavorable prognostic sign. In tuberculous meningitis, improvement in the course of the disease is accompanied by an increase in monocytic activity while the neutrophilic normalizes. In the majority of cases the monocyte reaction lasts longer than the clinical subsidence of the disease. In another series of investigations, the same author maintains that the monocytogram alone is not a reliable indicator of the reactivity of a child's organism. Regarding the pathogenesis of the newborn hemorrhagic disease, Soviet clinicians claim that not one of the blood factors (RBC, Hb., FI., reticulocytosis, erythroblasts, leucocytes, including stab, plasma proteins) is indicative of the presence of this disease.

Several authors published articles on the successful autotransfusions to women with extrauterine pregnancies who were operated on. The blood extravased during the operation and collected in the abdominal cavity was removed by means of small cups and poured into a blood bank through folded gauze soaked in 4% sodium citrate and counted on a ratio of sodium citrate to blood as 10 ml.: 100ml. As to the exchange transfusions, this was first introduced in Leningrad in 1951 and much later in Moscow. What Soviet hematology has achieved and where it stands is seen also by the fact that at the last Congress of the Europen Society of Hematology (1957) Russian hematologists did not give a single report. About the same time, on the occasion of the critical illness of a top Soviet Communist in Moscow, a consultant was taken there by plane, — a hematologist from the German Federal Republic!

The Soviet scientists were in no better form at the VIII International Congress on Hematology which took place in Tokyo, September 5-15, 1960. There they did not demonstrate one original idea, one original report, as judged by the account published in the *Herald of the AMS of USSR*, #2, 1961, pp. 70-78, by the participants and the prominent Soviet hematologists, Kassirsky, Alexeev and Bergholtz. In the said account it is mentioned: "As it is certain from the numerous publications, in experiments carried on in USSR, there has been success in isolating from the leucose tissues of man, a non-celled leucosogenic agent possessing many traits of a virus. The results of these investigations were briefly relayed in the statement of V. Bergholtz." Why "briefly" while on the same subject according to the same Soviet delegates American authors have in extenso and convincingly carried on their achievements in this field? The report read by the Soviet delegate, E. I. Atahanov, was on the subject of "The Hemogram in Chronic Enterocolitises." Further it said that the participation of the Soviet authors at the Congress and at the symposium on hematology was expressed in program reports. But which these reports were, besides the one mentioned above, is not pointed out by the authors of these very reports . . .

The Central Institute of Hematology and Transfusions has worked out a method of preparation of "thrombocytic mass" of fresh citrated blood which is used for its "hemostatic effect" in cases of blood discrasias (2-5 times every 3-5 days). The best effect has been found in Werlhof's *Disease and Hypoplastic Anemia.*

The only book of any note in hematology in USSR is a hematologic atlas by I. A. Kassirsky, a Soviet hematologist.

PHARMACOLOGY AND THERAPEUTICS

Therapeutics wear many of the characteristic features of Communist dialectic philosophy. Following are its peculiarities and some outmoded trends.

1. *Infections* open the door of illness and henceforth the organism's reactivity carries on a pathologic course of its own. The main goal of the therapeutist, therefore, should be to enhance the reactive defensive power of the organism.

2. *Vitamins,* especially Vitamin B and C, are considered of utmost importance in promoting the defensive power. The latter, more than any other is used in large doses in every case of more serious infection, malnutrition, disturbed metabolism, allergies, etc. Hypogalactia of the nursing mother is also treated by means of a diet rich in Vitamin C plus 300 mgs. daily for its insufficiency is considered one of the main causes of the failure. It "potentiates" penicillin and is given together with it in all infections. Vitamins are also called "biocatalizators." Recently L. N. Ignatova (Institute of Therapy) recommended B_{12} as a regulator of cholesterol in arteriosclerotic patients. Yes, one of the peculiarities of Soviet medicine is the vitaminomania.

The Soviet Union was perhaps the sole country which, as early as 1938 and 1939, held for two years consecutively the first All-Union conferences dedicated to the clinical application of vitamins. The transactions were published in two volumes. Of course those works (transactions) cannot be compared with such classical ones, for instance, as Bicknell-Prescott's (British) and those of numerous Americans on vitamins.

3. *"Biostimulators"* are widely used. By this is meant not only the vitamins but all kinds of physical therapies as well, such as Ultra-Violet radiation, in some cases X-ray radiation, sunlight, and climatotherapy in mountainous, field and sea areas. Diseases like tuberculosis, allergies of any kind, rheumatic fever in the subclinical stage or following sufficient improvement, asthma, etc., are reasons for forwarding patients to the so-called "Climatological Stations and Institutions" where they are subjected to programmed care for complete recovery in the course of one to six or more months.

To the group of biostimulators also belongs hemotherapy. Decades before, the I.M. introduction of blood (the patient's own blood or that of his closest relative,) was widely practiced. For the last decade this method has been less often applied and is more and more replaced by blood transfusions in small doses every four to six days for four to six consecutive times. Serum therapy in diphtheria is accompanied by hemotherapy to prevent serum sickness. However, Soviet medical literature, especially the pediatric, lacks articles revealing fear of hepatitis as a sequel to homotherapy, — a possibility of deep concern in the U.S.

Here belongs also the tissue therapy: — subcutaneous "burying" of a piece of animal tissue "ripened" by being kept for several days in special media. This method was practiced in many clinical entities like peptic ulcer, malnutrition, dysentery, etc. At first it was highly praised but more and more the enthusiasm is fading because as a "pan-therapy" it fails. In the successful instances they did not take into account the psychic effect, the time factor, etc.

4. As much *Aspirin* is used in pediatric practice in the U.S. (the cause of many disasters for children and infants) as pyramidon and allied are used in the USSR, but without the so much exaggerated and feared in the U.S. aggranulocytosis.

5. Many of the prescriptions are combinations prepared by the pharmacist. Soviet doctors have no fear of *polypragmasia* and prescriptions are augmented by unnecessary constituents. For instance, analeptics are prescribed for almost every case of illness with elevated temperature, lung complications or supposed "toxicity." Clinicians are recommending analeptics such as oleum camphoratum (10-20%) in doses even for children ranging from 2 to 3 years, of 3 to 6 cc. or more per 24 hours, given I.M. The therapeutic value of this was questioned and its use hated in the U.S. For besides being painful, it often is followed by complications. However, all this is well reconciled in the USSR by Pavlov's teaching.

6. They lack long acting antibiotic preparations of good quality like the Bicillin so effectively and conveniently used in the U.S. For this reason they apply penicillin in promptu and ad locum diluted in distilled water. At the time of each injection, 1% Procaine (Novoc.) or 1% Pyramidon sol. in the amount of ½ to 1 cc. is added in order to "delay" absorption. Thus, daily injections are reduced to two. This method, though unreliable, is widely practiced. As we mentioned previously, in particular cases they are still recommending that penicillin be injected from 4 to

6 or more times in 24 hours. This is clear-cut Communist barbarism, flavored with "scientific justifications."

7. Their antibiotics are only about one-fifteenth as many as are used in the U.S. As to their variety and quality, there is no comparison. Professor Roodnev, member of the Soviet Academy of Medicine, as late as the spring of 1956, in an extensive article published in *Medical Worker (Meditsinkii Rabotnik,)* bitterly criticized and complained about Soviet antibiotics, their ineffectiveness, unreliability as to their effect, less strength than shown on the labels, side effects and safety. This is the reason that no one in the Communist empire fully trusts the Soviet antibiotics or anything that is produced and exported by the USSR.

The writer of this series was hospitalized for 47 days in 1955. Following amputation of his legs, an infection appeared and was unsubdued for 42 days by means of Soviet Penicillin and Streptomycin. Then one of the doctors, a more kindly Communist, confidentially suggested to me that we find American Streptomycin. Thanks to friends, we received it the same day and five days later I was discharged.

Dr. M. Radionov, a non-Communist doctor-surgeon in Sofia, Bulgaria, of great help to the Communists during the time that they were subjected to imprisonment for anti-government activities, had prescribed Penicillin to a patient and uncautiously warned him to get the American product (at one time, 1956, it was available). Quite naively the patient cited the doctor's opinion to the pharmacist, a Communist, who immediately reported this to the government security and the doctor was deported to the deep Provintsia for six months. Apparently this situation has still not improved, because up to the present moment, cautiously they are complaining of the unreliability of their antibiotics.

Soviets do not have the most modern and important drugs. What they do have of them are used only at some of the central institutions. As to drug inventions, they have nothing in common with the corticosteroids, antihistamines, drugs against tuberculosis, tranquilizers, anticonvulsives, antimalarials and those used in the malignancies and endocrinology. All of these made epochs in the history of medicine and in the majority of cases are contributions of the U.S. medical science. In the early era of the Isoniazid, they copied and produced a similar anti-tuberculosis preparation of Fthivasid and there they remained with it up to the present moment. But they are dishonest as evidenced by such simple things as these: PAS was renamed PASK and proclaimed to be a "Soviet National Achievement" though it is not available at many peripheral institutions and antituberculosis dispensaries. (*Problems of T.B.*, #6, 1958.)

Further, they wrote, "Recently in our country's and foreign literature there have appeared communications regarding the successful treatment of ascaridosis and enterobiosis by means of derivatives of Piperazine." In fact, this treatment was known in Europe since 1950 and even earlier.

As to managing cardiac patients and the use of digitalis, the following is a classical example of Pavlovian-Nervism approach to a critical case. Simultaneously it shows the standard of a Soviet clinical institution of highest scientific rank.

Vete S., boy, 7, during the last 3½ years had suffered three attacks of atrial paroxysmal tachycardia. The fourth attack appeared following a fist blow in the abdomen (June 8, 1957). He was immediately hospitalized and unsuccessfully treated with Quinine, Digitalis and Vitamins. Within nine days the child had heart failure with cyanosis and a pulse of 200. He was transferred to the hospital of the Institute of Pediatrics in the city of Gorky. In a state of cyanosis, cardio and hepatomegaly, lung stasis, concurrent pneumonia, abdominal distension and insomnia, treatment with Quinine and Digitalis was renewed plus orally 0.03 gm of Pachicarpin b.i.d. and 1 cc. I.M. of 3% Sol. Acetylcholine twice with a seven day interval. However, there was no effect. In order to reduce the excitability of the subcortical centers and local interoreceptors of the heart muscle, Camphorated Bromine, Sodium Bromine and infusion of a grass, were given with no effect. Because of the precipitating trauma, subcapsular liver hematoma was admitted as being a continuous source of interoreceptive impulses for the cardio-vascular center. In order to block this pathological reflex, Novocain Iontophoresis of gangl. Stellate was performed. Two seances of this physiotherapy worsened the condition. Strophanthin and Magn. Sulf. for 5 days did not bring any effect. The increasing edema and ascites were fought by means of diuretics. On the fifth day in this hospital, total clouding of the left lung and interlobite in the right lung were found. The condition of the child was hopeless. On the 25th day after the onset of the attack the child was given 3 mg. of 2% Novocain (Procaine) in aqua distillata, I.M., introduced slowly. Result — abrupt discontinuation of the tachycardia.

Any senior medical student of Western Reserve University would wonder about this treatment based upon Pavlov's Nervism and applied to such a critically ill patient because of the following:

1.   The renewal of oral medication at the Institute of Pediatrics was wrong as the child already had heart failure and hepatomegaly and thus, absorption was impaired.

2.   Digitalis has been given by oral route and later Strophantin was not fully justified for reasons well known.

3.   No rapid digitalization was attempted parenterally.

4.   Quinine was not applied I.V.

5.   With respect to the supposed liver hematomes, no X-ray was used.

6.   The child was undertreated and the illness unduly prolonged. This led to the appearance of complications, to over-augmentation of treatment and its ineffectiveness.

We thus see how doctors of the highest ranking Institute of Pediatrics have become victims of theories which fail in practice and logics.

Rapid digitalization is now being cautiously considered by Professor B. E. Votchal (*Klinich. Meditsina,* #8, 1961). This method has been used in the U.S. for a long, long time.

Following is another example of the backwardness of Soviet clinicians. In *Klinicheskaya Meditsina* (#5, 1959,) there appeared two articles on the application of bee poison for the treatment of Radiculitises and Sciatica, (one by I. M. Sokolov and the other by K. F. Vladimirov). Docent (Professor) V. N. Kluchkov and A. A. Gabov from the Cathedra of Nervous Diseases at the Yaroslav Institute of Medicine make the following comments:

"Recently the clinics of nervous diseases at the Yaroslav Medical Institute have been carrying on systematic studies of the therapeutic values of bee poison in cases of lumbo-sacral radiculitises and neuritises of nervous Ischiadicus. We used the same preparation of bee poison as the above . . . authors. . . . The number of our patients was 21.

"Comparing the results from this treatment and those from the treatment by routine methods . . . we could not find appreciable advantages of the bee poison preparation diluted in oil. In this manner our data do not allow us to agree with the opinion of Vladimirov and Sokolov of the 'exclusively effective bee poison in the various forms of lumbo-ischiadic syndrome'."

These comments of Kluchkov-Gabov are published in #9 of *Klinicheskaya Meditsina*, 1960. Western doctors came across this drug in the thirties and after an initial enthusiastic acceptance it faded away in a few years. This experimentation of the Russians is a result either of insufficient information or of the pretension to "check" the claims of the capitalistic clinicians, though in that case a little late.

In tuberculosis which is difficult to manage, intra-bronchial introduction of antibiotics is practiced with good results, parallel with the rest of the complex treatments. By means of laryngeal syringe, a solution of streptomycin 200,000 units and Isoniazid 0.2, 3-4 ml. of 5% solution is introduced every day; a total of 10-40 instillations. It is claimed that the results are very good. The antibiotic substance "exercises" an effect on the entire organism.

The Fthivasid, a derivative of Isoniazid, is not mentioned as an anti-tuberculosis means in the pages of the Warsaw Collective Works on tuberculosis and published in 1956, (Editor — Professor Y. Nissevich). In a comparative classification by O. O. Makeeva, it is in third place, following Tubasid and Metasid, of course, according to their judgments.

Recently the Soviet medical press has been pointing out several new preparations against tuberculosis. For years they were proud of their Fthivasid which now proves to be more and more unsatisfactory because of its low blood levels. The new preparations are Etoxid, Ciclosterine, Duasid, and Methyl-fthivasid. However, they are not satisfied with these and are looking for new. With respect to Isoniazid, they recommend individualization and much larger doses, the idea for which we mentioned they have taken from the French.

In the complex treatment of pneumonia in children, the late Professor Maslov in his clinical lecture on pediatrics, recommended exposure to fresh air for 20-40 minutes several times each day.

In Soviet therapy, Sodium Bromide is still being used very, very much, starting with pediatrics and ending with psychiatry. Extensive research is also done with Bromine and its salts. This has deep roots in several specific Soviet realities. First the lack of other means, especially in the pretranquilizer era. Second, the concept that it is particularly effective in the normalization of the basic nervous processes — excitation and inhibition. Third, and most important, because Pavlov once said, "Fortunate is mankind for having such a blessed drug as Bromine," and at the time preceding his death, when his cortex failed to direct the vital processes, Pavlov himself resorted to using Bromine.

Soviet clinicians claim to have a new approach to the thrombo-embolic diseases and are endeavoring to prevent them. Surely the anticoagulants are such an approach. Before the application of anticoagulants to cases of myocardial infarction, lethality has been from 20% (Tareev) to 24% (Gelstein); after its use was introduced, lethality dropped to 7% and 3.3%. This therapy is applied in all cases where it is not contraindicated.

L. A. Koreisha says: "We can with confidence say that myocardial infarction, coronary disease, hypertension and so on do exist without signs of arteriosclerosis."

In his speech before the XV session of the AMS, its president, N. N. Blohin, pointed out new achievements in the field of therapy and drugs.

"The epidemiology of arteriosclerosis has been studied in four cities of the USSR (Tallin, Archangelsk, Ryazan and Stalinabad,) to determine the level of cholesterol in their population, to collect information with respect to their nutrition and the incidence of death from myocardial infarction. The data obtained shows a definite role in the nature of nutrition with respect to its fat content in the development of sclerosis of the coronaries.

"In the Institute of Therapy there has been constructed original apparatus allowing the separate study of the blood supply of an organism as a whole and of the heart of animals, and it was proved that the heart, humorally, is absolutely isolated from the rest of the organism and is linked with the latter only by means of the heart nerves. This apparatus allows the effects of the various stimulators and substances upon the coronary vessels to be studied without the distorting influences on the part of the somatic circulation." One is at a loss to place such an independence within the domain of Nervism.

Great interest is shown in the USSR to people's medicine as we have already briefly mentioned elsewhere. In the *Journal (Herald) of the AMS of USSR* (#8, 1960) there was published an extensive article "On the Study of the Experience of People's Medicine With Respect to the Application of Antibacterial Substances of Animal Origin." (A. A. Efremenko.) Concomitantly with relaying the history of the subject, Efremenko thus motivates his article and the interest in the matter of people's medicine:

"Little attention up to now has been paid to the bacteriostatic and bactericidal substances of animal origin, though the latter, being at a higher level of philogenetic development, ought to possess incomparably more perfect and more numerous devices for its defense against all kinds of pathogenic as well as saprophitic microorganisms. . . . The occurrence recently of a great variety of untoward effects after the application of antibiotics of mycotic origin dictates urgently the necessity of the study and research of new sources of biological antiseptics.

"Besides that . . . antibiotics inhibit immunogenesis, reduce phagocytosis and vitamins in the organism. (Vitamin C deficiency in animals is accompanied by a 25% decrease in the activity of lysosyme in the lungs, 37% in the spleen and 54% in the liver.)"

". . . Every day convince yourself that . . . really people's curative means cause no harm. (S. A. Smirnov.)

"The harmlessness of one of the most widespread people's means, — spider's web, — is experimentally confirmed by the work of G. P. Kirsanov just published (1959). It is greatly significant that these means have been and are being applied by the people of the entire world . . .

"In Egypt, 3,000 years ago, substances prepared from parts or fluids of animal origin were successfully applied. In 1595 in China a 52 volume pharmacopeia *Ben-Ghan-Moo* was published by Lee-Shee Chjen. Thirteen volumes were dedicated to the drugs of animal origin; there is pointed out the curative effect of the products of many animals from molusks and insects to man. Many of them, it is claimed, have effect against infectious diseases, — dysentery, typhoid fever, malaria, TB and so on. In the famous *Cannon of Medical Science* of Avicenna, out of the 811 medicines described in the second book, 125 are of animal origin."

By experimental and clinical study of the remedies of people's medicine, many of the facts stressed before find theoretical substantiation. Thus it has been known for a long time that —

"Egg white and saliva favorably help in curing sores, wounds, cuts, burns, and so on.

Egg white was applied in ancient ophthalmology.

Egg white application to wounds and sores has been recommended by many authors, throughout history: pure, or egg white plus olive oil.

People have been treating wounds with saliva — human, or by being licked by dogs.

Saliva has been applied in the treatment of the eyes, when ill or prophylactically.

In Iran they collect the tears and apply them only when all other means have failed, so precious and costly they have been considered.

I. I. Manuhin (1911) subjected the leucocytes to lysis, thus obtaining antibacterial substances which he used for the treatment of infectious diseases.

Caucasus' foresters apply bone marrow, considering it to have great antibactericidal properties.

Horse's spleen bactericidal activity has been studied by A. I. Kondratev (1896). He prepared extracts of it which were able to prevent tetanus in mice subsequently subjected to infection with tetanus.

The skin of animals and man possess antibactericidal effect as evidenced by the fact that people apply fresh animal skins for treatment of wounds, sores or burns.

A. A. Pervushina (1951) and K. M. Lebedeva (1957) proved that man's skin possesses the property of killing microbes, but this depends also on other factors.

Fish tissues and organs have a curative effect.

For hemostatic reasons spider's web has effectively been applied by the people.

Since remote times people have been applying animal fats for treatment of sores, burns, decubital sores and others."

A. A. Efremenko, author of the detailed article, concludes it with the hope that the study of animal antibiotics may result in the discovery of new means for the treatment of surgical, dermatological and gynecological illnesses. Yes, if Western and American scientists discover such. He mentions that the article was written when it had become known that G. P. Kirsanov had established that spider's web possesses antibiotic properties of wide spectrum lasting two years. The interest of the Russians in this field has been very great for the last 25 years. We have given in detail the above reviewed article in the hope that some drug firms or other institutions in the U.S. might find it useful. If any one is interested further, we will be glad to translate it in full for him.

This 1961 academical year, academician-Professor S. V. Anichkov was awarded for a series of works on the pharmacology of the CNS.

Continuing to quote from President N. N. Blohin's speech, he said:

"New complex methods of treatment of Acute Rheumatic Fever were worked out by means of applying hormonal and pyrazolol preparations. On the way are measures regarding the prophylaxis with bicillin against the relapses of acute rheumatic fever and also measures with respect to the prophylaxis of rheumatismal diseases of children of pre-school and school age.

"During the period we are accounting for, new drugs have been offered for the treatment of cardio-vascular diseases and among them Chlorazine is the preparation possessing selective coronaro-dilatative action." *(Herald, AMS of USSR, #9, 1961.)*

On January 12, 1962, the *Akron Beacon-Journal* carried the following AP dispatch out of London:

"Rush Drugs For Red Scientist. — A British Comet jetliner flew to Moscow today with a consignment of five drugs for Professor Lev Landau, a top Soviet physicist gravely ill in a Russian hospital. The drugs are designed to prevent fluid accumulating in the brain and to combat pneumonia. The 53-year-old physicist developed pneumonia and was reported unconscious days after suffering severe head injuries in an automobile wreck."

This case refers to British drugs. And what British drugs and medicine are, compared to American, we pointed out elsewhere the opinion of prominent Britons.

There are in the Soviet Union 280 scientific institutes, of which a dozen are carrying on research in the field of internal, cardio-vascular, nutritional diseases and in the field of pharmaceutics, pharmacology and therapy. In the U.S. in 1960, the National Institute of Health alone tested 50,000 potential cancer-fighting drugs. And there are 3200 private laboratories producing drugs. They are carrying on the greatest research that has ever been performed in any nation on earth. Three thousand and two hundred laboratories with their staffs, — free, undisturbed and conscientious, pursuing their original goals, methods, ambitions and plans. Their achievements are awarded Nobel Prizes

and are praised throughout the world; they are pre-
ferred more than any other product; people under
Communist yoke, even the academicians themselves,
look for the American medicines and follow the American methods and ideas. The voices raised recently
asking the U.S. government to interfere in the research
by abolishing the patent rights mean nothing but a
step backward with the potential of definite degres-
sion. For we must admit that the violent adherence
to the teaching of Pavlov may be a perverse reaction
on the part of those who are enslaved, humiliated and
despairing under Communism and who have the right
to wander along the fields of optimistic philosophy of
which Pavlov provides vast opportunities, on the one
hand and to compensate for the poverty of Soviet
medical inventive realities on the other hand.

So, Soviet medicine and Soviet medics and academicians are very pretentious and boastful. They
claim that their science and political ideas are posi-
tivistic and materialistic. In fact, they are very speculative and talkative; they carry on tremendous research,
which we cannot maintain is a waste. But this is all.
The productivity and the fruitful completion of the
research are always a distance from them. And we
should never forget that they have free and vast access
to the American scientific trends and achievements.
This is of tremendous scientific and economic significance. At the same time, Americans are generally
unaware, or aware very little and too late, of the
developments of Soviet medicine.

The writer of this work never came across an impressive Soviet text book on Pharmacology and Therapeutics. But he has used several handbooks of that nature.

They all retain the fashion of compendiums which were popular 30-40 years ago.

While this is true regarding Soviet Science of Pharmaco-Therapy as seen in those booklets, the American works of T. Sollmann, Goodman and Gilman and of Best and Taylor basically remain unique especially as a combined source.

PHYSICAL THERAPY

No doubt, organized physical therapy is resorted to in the USSR more than in any other country in the world. The other peculiarity is that it is not provided as a private enterprise but all is maintained by the government within the free health service. Besides Soviet medics have a mania for the use of physical therapy.

There are several fields of physical therapy to which patients are assigned according to their illness and the phase of it. In this respect, children are given a most thorough care.

Climatotherapy. Scattered, and located at suitable climatological sites in the country, especially around the Black Sea shores, are the so-called Climatic Stations or Climatic Curative Stations. Some of them are strictly specific, others serving several categories of patients. Patients whose "body reactivity" is lagging or is inactive, in whom various illnesses are protracted and who need "biogenic stimulation" are always sent to such stations for three to six months and even more. The following types of patients deserve special mention.

1. Tuberculous lymphadenitis, scrophulosis, pulmonary tuberculosis in the subsiding phase, bone tuber-

culosis in which the nervous system is conspicuously involved (intoxicated), tuberculous pleurisy in the recovery phase and after complete resorption.

2.   Rheumatic fever patients in the post acute phase when the Sed. rate has considerably or completely normalized.   In other words, when the patient is in the so-called remission or inter-relapsing period of the illness.

3.   Allergic patients, first among them being the Asthmatics.

At the International symposium on the problem of treatment of lung tuberculosis patients with resistant BK toward three fundamental anti-tuberculous preparations, the USSR did not find any recognition of even their much commended preparation of Fthivasid. Professor N. A. Shmelev attempted to attract the attention of the delegates to this drug because of the presence on its side branch of the vanilin radical which according to him secures prolonged retention in the organism, and more stable though lower concentration in the blood than the standard drugs.   This was not accepted.

September 20-23, 1962 in Bulgaria-Varna there was an International symposium dedicated to skeletal tuberculosis.   The only new element which was discussed was the extirpation of intra and extra joint tuberculous foci insusceptible to healing and under antibacterial protection; that at the climatic stations patients benefit not only from the climate or from one sort of physical therapy but from several of them at one time, including physical exercises (training in breathing).   This handling of the patients is characteristic of the first two groups also.

Hydrotherapy comprises the various sorts of natural

or artificially prepared mineral water, hot and warm. To obtain treatment, the patients reside near such sources of water, either in hotels or communes, the latter consisting in part of specially built hydrotherapeutic institutions (stations). The time of treatment varies from twenty days to two or more months.

Hydrotherapy is combined with *iontophoresis; electricity;* powerful *water currents* which produce the effect of a blow upon the muscles, joints and bones; *friction* upon the skin of the whole body, or in parts with a rough piece of cloth soaked in cold water; *alternate exposure* of the whole body to cold and hot showers, etc.

Radiation therapy consists of X-ray treatment; UVR treatment; exposure to direct sun rays; diatherm and ultratherm (ultrasonic). Every hospital or clinic is equipped with several of these means. With doctors who have limited therapeutic pharmaceutical means and with patients who are too pretentious, very, very much resort is had to all possible sorts of physical therapy. Conditions are often miserable, some of the apparatus almost always out of order, and the public is in bitter discontent.

Massages. Every "united hospital" has on the staff trained massagists who serve the hospitalized patients and O.P.s, as well as those confined to their homes but who need such treatment.

In the USSR a remarkable number of intriguing text books on physical therapy exist.

Diet Therapy and Nutrition

In nutrition, Soviet medicine abounds with the most original ideas. The fundamental principles of Soviet science of nutrition and diet therapy are based on the philosophy of dialectic materialism and Soviet version of biology. Food is considered as a part of the environment with which animal and human organisms have a most intimate relation, since it is being ingested and becomes a constituent of the internal medium of the organism. And as the latter is inseparable from the environment, and it constitutes one whole with the environment, it is understandable that by changing the environment, that is, the food mainly, we can, say the Communists, induce and control changes in the organism.

Pavlov postulated that "the most important link of animal organism with surrounding nature is that through certain chemical substances, which continuously enter into the constitution of the same organism, that is, the link through the food."

These aspects are made clearer by the concept of I. P. Razenkov, one of the foremost contemporaries and disciples of Pavlov: "In the qualitative and varying nutrition, we possess a powerful factor by whose help we can intentionally enforce or weaken the functions and the trophics of the tissues, organs, systems and the organism as a whole." In nutrition of the organism, he says, the same interrelations occur as those in bacterial toxic agents. Sechenov maintained that "to trace the fate of the nutritional substances in the organism is to recognize life itself." Feeding, therefore, should not be looked upon as something routine, of a definite pattern, mechanical and only as a means of life, but as an adjustment of the organism to the surrounding environment in order that it may withstand those factors which are unfavorable. And all these and the rest of the vital processes and the mechanisms that are realizing them are directed, correlated and controlled by the central nervous system. That is the philosophy of Nervism.

Tareev maintains that the satiated man, in contradistinction from the hungry one, is characterized not only by different blood chemistries, but with different sensitivity of the analyzers and different nervous activity as well. People have proverbs concerning the hungry man, such as "hungry eyes get no sleep, hungry ears do not hear, hungry man has irritable nerves, hunger is a bad counselor." Y. A. Yakolinsky points out that experimental animals' nervous activity differs when they are fed with animal protein from when they are fed plant protein. From a biochemical and evolutionary point of view, animal food, that is, animal protein, has contributed much to the higher evolution of man's brain development and function. Such is Engels' opinion and it seems to have scientific foundation.

N. I. Krasnogorsky found that following feeding, the excitability of the brain cortex decreases, while about four hours later it acquires the maximal excitability. This means that frequent feeding of children is harmful in the sense that the higher nervous activity is impaired to the degree of impairing the entire health, defense, etc. People consider it a bad omen when anyone eats quite frequently or abundantly. Misfortunes occur to such men. In the light of Pavlov's teaching, as interpreted by Krasnogorsky, any accident to such a man becomes explainable and should not be regarded with superstition.

Upon these materialistic-dialectic concepts, or as they call them, "the higher stage of Darwinism," is constructed one of the best, from a practical point of view, textbooks of Dietotherapy by M. I. Pevzner,

Foundations of Therapeutic Nutrition. Pevzner belongs to the oldest generation of doctors under Communism. He is the Director of the Moscow Institute of Therapeutic Nutrition. His textbook is a voluminous work containing extensive scientific information, mostly of foreign origin. The various types of nutrition are outlined as indicated, by the various clinical entities. This work seems superior to M. G. Wohl's *Dietotherapy and Clinical Application of Modern Nutrition,* Saunders Company, Philadelphia, Pa. The latter's scientific value is very high but it is a product of sixty contributors, not as practical, and somewhat mechanistic. Pevzner's work is a realization of himself alone and besides is much more specific and detailed and gives a more complete and systematic idea of nutrition in health and disease.

In order to illustrate what is meant by "dialectical" nutrition, we will point out some of the diets of tuberculous patients (children) as outlined by Pevzner.

In deficient combative reactivity of the organism: Proteins of high quality, three to four grams per kg. of body weight; fats one and one-half gm. per kg. of body weight; carbohydrates, just enough to meet the necessary daily energetic needs, sufficient to spare the proteins but not to produce deposition of fats; Vitamins A, B, C, D. Vitamins A and D in physiological doses. Vitamin E as an anti-oxydant, if not contraindicated because of other medical reasons, should be taken in the quantities contained in whole wheat bread. Corresponding diets are given for tuberculous children with hyperfunction of the thyroid gland (mostly girls in adolescence;) such with phenomena of considerable destruction of focal tuberculous lesions; those with distinctly shown allergic diathesis; those with tendencies towards serositis, exudations and trans-udations; children with predominant manifestations on the part of the digestive system, such as poor appetite, vomiting and dyspepsia. Pevzner outlines these particular diets with the belief that even the constitution can be changed and so the effect aimed at, attained. For regardless of modern progress and high effectiveness of the antibacterial agents, it is an unconditional maxim to Soviet clinicians to consider of primary importance the reactivity of the macroorgan-ism and this is determined, first of all, they claim, by environment, one of the most important constituents of which is food. Hospitals in USSR use over a dozen different types of diets. In all cases of active infec-tion, especially tuberculosis, salt and abundant carbo-hydrates are considered by Russian clinicians to be unfavorable for the defensive capacities of the organ-ism because of their property to retain more water in the macroorganism and thus decrease its resistance and combative power.

There is no doubt that in all fields of public health Soviet medicine has achieved tremendous successes. But with respect to nutrition, the country is lacking the variety and abundance so characteristic of the West and especially the U.S. The Satellites, however, are in a poorer, even desperate condition of supply because all products of quality are exported to the USSR at prices which are government secrets. But even so, the vast Russian masses do not see much of the imported foods.

The winter vegetable and fruit supply for the Soviet people, with their children, consists mainly of sour cabbage, potatoes and sour apples, and this season in the USSR lasts for more than six months. During the summer, people rarely see a half of a tomato in a week, not to mention other vegetables and fruits. When they appear on the market they are not a product of those who are building missiles but, as we said, of the "satellites." Bulgaria, for instance, is the main supplier to the USSR of these items at a "brotherly cost." People in my country were making fun of the Russian medicine and biology, for having established that the best food for the Bulgarians is cabbage, while the worst, — cheese, meat, eggs, milk and fruits, — are exported to the USSR!

Professor O. P. Molchanova, one of the most renowned experts in public health and nutrition, recognizes the nutritional conditions in the USSR as follows:

". . . We may consider that in the USSR the physiological norms of nutrition per capita of the population have already been attained, the quantity of calories being approximately 3,000. However, the correlation of the nutritional substances and the quantity of the full value protein is far from the physiological norms of nutrition. . . . In many republics consumption of carbohydrates is much higher and there is not a sufficient amount of animal protein." *(Herald of the Academy of Medical Sciences of the USSR, #9, 1961.)*

In the resolution of the All-Soviet Union Conference on Nutrition which we mentioned before, it is said that "The control should be intensified in order that milk and other products of quality can be secured for children." *(Pediatria, #7, 1957, p. 104.)* Of course, such language as the above of Molchanova is an overall platitude, for no one dares to say more.

Recently the Institute of Nutrition elaborated physiological norms for six age groups of children, four adult groups depending on the nature of their labor, and two old age groups (up to 65 and more). With respect to the so-called curative-prophylaxis nutrition, the Institute of Nutrition in 1960 revised all of the ratios used in the various sections of industry and scientifically indicated changes were introduced. Nutrition as necessitated by the new field of cosmic flight has also been determined.

At the conference of the Government scientific-research Institute of Vitamilology, G. Y. Korpliakova reported of a decrease of vitamin B_6 and Niacin in TB patients who are subjected to prolonged anti-bacterial treatment; L. I. Noozberg reported an analogous phenomenon regarding B_1; V. A. Karmilova reported of endogenic Niacin hypovitaminosis in acute rheumatic fever patients; M. C. Useva reported on disproteinemia in children having rickets; L. I. Ermilova reported how the large doses of vitamin D affect the Ca in the blood of rats. She recommends the combined medication of D and A as calcification of soft tissues is not produced even if Vitamin D is given in large doses; V. F. Gorvat reported that toxicoses of pregnancy, having taken place even in the earlier stages affects Niacin in the breast milk and as a result of that — affects the organism of the infant. (T. N. Haustova, *Problems of Protection of Motherhood and Childhood*, March, 1962, p. 89.)

Professor O. P. Molchanova writes: "From the work carried on at the Institute of Nutrition, it has become certain that in the case of choline — protein deficiency, fatty degeneration of the liver may ensue with subsequent cirrhosis of the liver and even the appearance of non-malignant as well as cancerous neoplasms."

(Similar observations were published twenty years ago by South African, British, Indian and American authors — A.N.)

"In persons working at night, a slowing down of the pulse, decrease of BP and body temperature is observed, viz., these phenomena which occur during regular night sleep. Therefore, the organism experiences great tension and as a prophylactic measure the organization of a rational nutrition may be recommended for persons working at night." The lady-professor then goes on to describe in detail the nutritional elements and the regulation of the nutrition of such persons. This all sounds a little ridiculous in the countries of abundance and great variety of foods. Professor Debré showed fifteen years ago that even little children, left to their own choice, pick up the foods out of a variety, meeting the physiological demands.

INTERNAL MEDICINE

This field is totally dominated by Pavlov's teaching of Nervism. It is the widest medical field, focusing every branch of medicine, so it represents, better than any other, the nature, the advance and the possibilities of Soviet medicine. It is therefore justifiable here to discuss more the aplomb of Pavlov at this discipline of medical science.

There are two main areas in which Soviet internists are attempting to demonstrate the scientific validity of Pavlov's teaching of Nervism as it is understood by them. These areas are the peptic ulcer disease, as they call this illness, because they are of the strong opinion that it is an ailment of the organism as a whole, and the hypertensive disease, also thought to be an over-all nervous disturbance of the organism. Both are looked upon as the result of the disorder of the two fundamental processes of the brain cortex, — of excitation and of inhibition. Of course, this imbalance of the excitation and inhibition, with the nervous system being the controlling, directing and adjusting organ of the entire organism, constitutes the basic philosophy of Nervism, and they underlie the entire pathology of man. The therapy of the latter, therefore, consists of preventing the imbalance or of restoring the balance between the two processes.

I. *Peptic Ulcer Treatment.*

Treatment is confined to inducing sleep and restoring the equilibrium between inhibition and excitation. They give large doses of Phenobarbital sufficient to bring about deep sleep for 20 to 30 days. The patient is awakened only to eat. The results? Nil and more. In recent years the writer has not found one article in the Soviet medical journals with reference to this method and its reliability. The adherence to the diet remains the universal pattern, while other methods of treatment are attempted. This is apparent from the following excerpts.

"Up to the present there are not a few debatable and unresolved questions in the problem of peptic ulcer disease. Our work is the summary of the results of the study of 3284 patients treated in the therapeutic and surgical departments of the stationary (hospital) . . . 50% of the patients were observed by the authors in person. . . . A careful study of the history of 400 patients showed that in 211 of them the etiological factor had not been discovered, in 9 there had been a nervous distress, in 14 long nervous strain (tension,) in 29 irregular eating, in 21 unbalanced nutrition, in 36 chronic gastritis, in 31 chronic appendicitis, in 19 chronic cholecystitis . . ."

With respect to the therapy of peptic ulcer disease, the authors go on to say, "the new means of treatment in recent years by our fatherland's and foreign authors (hormones, ganglion blocking preparations, new spasmolitic means and alkalies, vitamin U (?), antibiotics, various combinations of sleep inducing preparations, biogenic stimulators) did not substantially change the immediate and the remote results in comparison with the 'classic' anti-ulcer treatment (. . . Gordon, Boas, von Noorden and others,) adherents to which we are." (A. R. Zlotopolsky, candidate of medical sciences, A. I. Hozanov and A. A. Zgun, Moscow, "Some Questions of the Clinics and the Treatment of Peptic Ulcer Disease," read at the meeting of "Gastroenterological Section of the Moscow Association of Therapy," November 4, 1959, *Klinicheskaya Meditsina*, #2, 1961.)

There is only one reference to Pavlov, — "The various combinations of sleep preparations." If we accept a priori that the etiology is presumably Pavlovian regardless of the cases enumerated, then why the resort to the treatment by means of the old "classical" method of diet and ultimately of surgery? This defeat of Pavlovism as practiced by the Soviet academicians is further evidenced by the complete lack of any reference to Pavlov and Nervism in the review of the achievements of Soviet medicine in connection with the forty years following the Revolution, and by omitting Pavlovism on the occasion of the XXII Congress of the Communist Party. Here is the newest evidence:

"Though in the clinics (on Internal Diseases — author's note) great significance is attributed to the nervous factors in the origin of myocardial infarction, we do not possess experimental data confirming it up to the present time." — N. N. Blohin, President of the AMS of USSR, *Vestnik (Herald) of the Academy of Medical Sciences of USSR*, #9, 1961.

The only mention of Pavlov in the lengthy speech of President Blohin is with respect to the Pavlovist Physiologists and this is to criticize, not praise them. (See section on Physiology.)

II. *Hypertensive Disease (Essential Hypertension)*

This illness as explained on the grounds of Nervism, was extensively dealt with by the late Professor G. F. Lang of Leningrad, in his excellent work dedicated to this illness. It is built upon extensive personal material and on a wide use of foreign literature. The basic concept is the teaching of Nervism, the substantiation of which is derived from the hypertension in monkeys which Lang and his co-workers induced by means of artificially caused neuroses. We know that psychoneuroses are caused by an enormous variety of factors to which the organisms respond, more or less, with individual specificity; with a clinical picture and response to treatment which is strictly specific and corresponding, no doubt, to the underlying biophysiological processes which are primarily biochemical.

To explain, therefore, that all this derives from one single pathophysiological mechanism, — the disequilibrium between the excitation and inhibition is impossible and one cannot accept it.

Finally, we are still in the dark with respect to the actual role of the activating system of the brain which became known in recent years. We may admit the possibility that the excitation and the inhibition may be out of balance, not primarily of themselves but as a result of the disorder of the activating system. What role does this system play in arousing a disturbance of those two fundamental processes? Is it a product or a cause of other underlying disturbance? These and many other questions are still unanswered and our reservations and the failure of Soviet clinicians are conceivable.

At present, Soviet internists and clinicians are in general preoccupied with research on the causes and the treatment of the vascular diseases. But the Committee of Cardio-Vascular Pathology at the Academy of Medical Sciences finds lack of unity in the work of the institutes, lack of definite aims, and a very small number of long term observations.

While there is nothing concrete for the Soviet internists to boast about, recently in a published monograph they claim that they have priority in describing a number of clinical syndromes. Which they are is uncertain.

One of the internists of greatest renown in USSR is the late G. F. Lang whom we mentioned elsewhere and whose work on Hypertension remains classical in Soviet medical literature. However, he who was an excellent cardiologist maintained (in 1938) that only five to ten percent of the patients with myocardial infarction can go back to work, while as late as 1954, T. B. Karenevskaya postulated that this percentage reaches the figure of 70! A. L. Miasnikov is another outstanding internist. He is the author of a good number of scientific works and books. A characteristic of his medical erudition we find in the following example. In the October, 1960, issue of *Klinicheskaya Meditsina*, comments are published with respect to the classification by Miasnikov of the sudden deaths of patients with arteriosclerosis of the coronary arteries. These are the comments of N. M. Dimenteva who criticizes Miasnikov for not saying anything in his classification regarding the so-called hidden, unmanifested and uncomplained of forms of coronary sclerosis prior to the sudden death. The author concludes with the remark that the percentage of those cases is as high as 42. It is difficult for the reader to understand how it is possible for an internist of academical rank and considered to be one of the two or three most outstanding Soviet clinicians, to omit to take into consideration such clinical facts as are known even by lay people.

Before the Fifteenth session of the AMS of the USSR, dedicated to the XXII Congress of the Communist Party of USSR, the same academician, A. L. Miasnikov, read a report on "Ways of Finding Means and Methods for the Treatment and Prophylaxis of Cardio-Vascular Diseases." He spoke on three illnesses, Hypertonic Disease, Arteriosclerosis, and Insufficiency of the Coronaries. In ending his discussion on Hypertonic Disease (Essential Hypertension — Author's Note) he says:

"Recently we created a combined preparation, conditionally designated as Depressin, and consisting of

Hypothiazid	25 mgs.
Reserpin	0.1 mg.
Diabasol	0.02 Gm.
Nembutal	0.05 Gm.

The first results obtained, thanks to this, as it seems to us, very good curative preparation, are given in Table 3."

In this Table 3 Miasnikov gives the number of patients, 136, to whom the preparation has been applied. This number, of course, is very insufficient for conclusions in a report before such a body as the Academy in session dedicated to the Communist Party. Moreover, the preparation of Depressin consists of drugs invented by the West and the U.S. scientists. Miasnikov has only made a combination of them and christened it.

Further on, based on experimental and clinical observations at the Institute of Therapy, its Director-Professor, academician A. L. Miasnikov, proposes the following preparation of Delipin containing

Ascorbic acid	300 mgs.
Methionin	300 mgs.
Vitamin B_6	50 mgs.
(or Niacin	50-100 mgs.)
Luminal	20 mgs.

This combination is intended to prevent the formation of arteriosclerosis, including that of the coronaries. He explains that the constituents act upon the various phases and rings of the pathological process.

Quite recently Soviet scientists undertook a wide and detailed study of the causes and the prevention of arteriosclerosis and first of all that of the coronary arteries. In this study it is claimed that:

"In the process of being worked out are new methods of the diagnosis of the cardio-vascular diseases; in particular there has been designed a new variant of precordial reocardiograph to provide a separate study of the contractive function of heart ventricles.

"With respect to the studies of the immunogenesis of acute rheumatic fever, carried on in the Institute of Rheumatism, there are methods worked out for the immunological diagnostics of acute rheumatic fever, non-specific arthritises and other collagenoses. In the blood serum of these patients a specific antigen was found."

A book on Phonocardiography appeared a year ago (1960), its author being a woman cardiologist, L. M. Fitileva.

E. M. Tareev is another internist, the author of what is no doubt the best and almost the only Soviet textbook on internal diseases. It is a thick, one volume book of ordinary format whose first edition appeared in 1951 or 1952. Compared with the classical textbooks on internal diseases such as Osler-Christian's, French Vidal's series, German Mehring's volumes, and the old but excellent work of Strumpell, Tareev's does not equal any of them.

At the Eighth All-Union Conference of Soviet Internists (June 29-July 2, 1955) again Tareev read a report on the subject of "General Questions on Applying Antibiotics in the Clinics." A great number of those present commented. Following are some of the comments.

G. N. Chekulaev: "The classification which Tareev proposes, consisting of three main groups is not original, as in American literature an analogous classification exists." *(Works of the Eighth All-Union Conference of the Internists, MEDGIZ, Leningrad Division, 1956, p. 69.)*

L. A. Varshamov: "It is necessary to take into consideration that the material of the report of Professor Tareev is based, to a great extent upon, in particular, American literature." (Ibid., p. 71.)

A. M. Sigal: "Many of the cases mentioned by him (Tareev) regarding the side effects of the antibiotics are widely described in the American literature." (Ibid., p. 66.)

It is not insignificant that up to the present time the articles published in *Vestnik Academii Meditsinkih Nauk of USSR (Herald of the Academy of Medical Sciences of USSR)* are given without summaries in any foreign language as well as (with some exceptions) without bibliography. The names of foreign authors quoted, most of the time are spelled in the Russian alphabet. This is neither neglect nor poverty nor ignorance of foreign languages, for most of the other journals regularly give summaries in a foreign language and bibliography with the original spelling of the names of the authors. The above cited publication of the Academy of Medical Sciences of USSR serves first of all the academicians and the highest ranking scientists, and is published in an edition of 3,000 copies. We leave it to the reader to draw his own conclusions as to the motivations which have driven Soviet academicians to disregard the elementary rule and faithfulness in dealing with science. Of course they do not miss carrying on the ideological warfare against the West. Another indication is that with 400,000 doctors and thousands of institutions, the Academy's scientific organ is issued in 3,000 copies!

In *Klinicheskaya Meditsina*, #2, 1961, the leading editorial article is dedicated to the pure ideology of Communism by means of discussing Engels' dialectical philosophy in medicine as counterposed to the non-dialectical Western world and its science. This shows the real ideological image of Communist scientists which is one of dishonesty and warfare against the free world, — from which image Western and American scientists and doctors greatly differ, and whose meaning they are ignoring.

PEDIATRICS

Child health and pediatrics have absorbed the greater part of the efforts of the Soviet medical profession, related institutions and factors. The work done in the past and at present, and the money spent, are beyond estimation, especially the former. Great is the number of founders, inspirers and leaders of Soviet-Russian pediatrics. For decades there have been two centers of pediatric science as theory and practice, one in Moscow and the other in Leningrad. No doubt the first place belongs to the latter which was led by a highly gifted clinician, Dr. M. C. Maslov, author of several books on pediatrics and professor at the Leningrad Medical Institute (School). He died not long ago.

In Leningrad also work two other eminent pediatricians, academicians and professors, A. F. Toor and M. G. Danilevich, an infectionist. Both are authors of textbooks and the latter's book especially, on Infectious Diseases, is widely known and highly valued. At Leningrad also is Professor N. I. Krasnogorsky, pediatrician, dedicated to research in pediatrics based on the teaching of I. P. Pavlov. A few only of the top ranking women-pediatricians work in Leningrad, the great majority being in Moscow.

These men, together with the Moscow representatives and leaders in pediatrics are the propelling force and at the same time, the main tool in the hands of the Party for the tremendous successes in the field of child welfare.

In USSR there are about 60,000 pediatricians, almost all women. In the U.S. there are about 9,000 pediatricians of which only 5,600 possess licensure. Soviet pediatricians theoretically should be well prepared since they, as in all other specialties, early in the medical course are profiled for the pediatric field.

The achievements are really great in comparison with the situation before the revolution. An unusual number of various conferences dedicated to child welfare are held locally, all-Union, even for the entire Communist empire. Everyone of them is a tremendous pledge, — a crusade. The end result of this is the achievements: considerable reduction in morbidity and mortality, and unbelievable increase in hospital beds, kindergartens and sanitoriums for children. However, it is difficult for the reader to judge correctly by the comparative percentage figures which are similar to the ones they use in the military field. The progress and achievements of Soviet pediatrics and of public health are nevertheless unquestionable.

However, Soviet pediatric specialty has still to deal with many problems which are forgotten in the West and especially in the U.S. Such is the case with tuberculosis, pertussis, tetanus, diphtheria, rickets, malnutrition, acute disorders of the digestive system, and others, not to speak of the primitiveness of vast area of the Communist conglomerate empire.

As to the clinical field, there is nothing interesting in Soviet pediatrics. For originalities there we have to look along the Pavlovian lines. But at the present stage of Pavlov's teaching as it is advocated and interpreted by his "disciples," it is hard to give ourselves an approximate account of its real achievements in pediatrics. While we have enough proof to doubt its significance in the clinics, in respect to education, social pathology and pedagogy it reveals promising aspects. The merit here mainly belongs to N. I. Krasnogorsky who gives us his findings regarding little children and their capability of forming conditioned reflexes. As we know, those reflexes are the key to all learning and the main bulk of the higher nervous activity. We present a summary of them.

Little children form conditioned reflexes in stages. First they are indifferent or show orienting reflex; after repetition, their reaction becomes established; still later, the established reflex blocks any other brain activity and finally it becomes automatic (habitual). Conditioned reflexes are generally formed quickly; they are extremely stable; babies, from the very first moment after birth, are capable of forming them; outer stimulators to the newborn are very strong and therefore his cortex becomes easily exhausted and this leads to physiological sleep; so, first of all, the prematures do; little children's cortex is weak and because of that they show tendencies toward generalized reactions, stimulation easily reaches the lower brain areas and convulsions arise with ease; synthetic capacity is great, especially in the second year; sleep conquers the most exhausted cells, — first those of hearing and speech analyzers; physiological sleep (without medication) exercises powerful curative effect; fresh air has an excellent sleep effect; formation of conditioned reflexes diminishes as nutrition of children worsens; there is a direct parallelism between arrest of growth and decrease of formation of conditioned reflexes; higher nervous activity is highly dependent on the hormonal system. All those facts have been known to pedagogy for centuries, and as well to intelligent laymen and parents.

Moscow's *Pediatria*, #9, 1958, published an article dedicated to Krasnogorsky on the occasion of his fiftieth year of scientific activity and seventy-fifth year of age. With the exception of the conventional praises and biographical data, that in 1935 he had been awarded for his monograph "Development of the Teaching of the Physiological Activity of Children's Main Brain," and that in 1958 he had submitted for print a monograph on "The Higher Nervous Activity of the Healthy and Sick Child," strangely enough no other concrete merits were pointed out! This and worse occurred to him on the occasion of the XXII Party Congress, where no mention was made of his name, and no regard for new achievements. Pavlovism was generally ignored and the Pavlovists were not praised but rather reprimanded because of lack of worthy contributions.

By the way, about a year ago I met an American, closely related to Western Reserve University. It is a curious observation that while we were commenting on Soviet science and physiology, he recalled that Krasnogorsky was on the staff of the University before World War II; he had done his utmost to get his wife and daughter out of the USSR in order that he would never have to return to his country; he did not succeed and had no other choice but to return to the USSR. However, Krasnogorsky is an honest, unservile and dedicated scientist differing much from the majority of other academicians-scientists.

As to the application of Pavlov's teaching in modern pediatric clinics, here are some of the failures. I. V. Kazhansky and V. N. Ananeva (1958) treated children who were ill with acute dysentary, with enemas of 1% novocain plus 0.6 sodium chloride, aiming at blocking the local interoreceptors. Simultaneously the rest of the complex treatment was carried on. They had a control group. Result — no difference. V. A. Novikova (1958) published an article regarding children ill with chorea and affected heart, and their treatment with interrupted sleep (induced by means of sleep drugs). The children were followed for five years. Conclusion: "Treatment with sleep cannot be considered as something contenting and basic by itself." Children suffering from anorexia which have become strongly conditioned in Pavlov's sense, when an attempt is made at disinhibiting them by means of taking their attention away in time of feeding, show a stabilization of the negative conditioned reflex of anorexia.

In a review of forty years of children's psychoneurology, nothing is pointed out as an achievement in pediatrics in Pavlov's field. It is claimed, however, that Soviet psychoneurology has first admitted the possibility of schizophrenia starting in early childhood, a boast again ungrounded.

How far and by which method the favorable aspects of Pavlov's teaching may be applied in the every day life of children and in dealing with children is very much an open question. For even in USSR we do not see a convincing and wide introduction of Pavlov's teaching in the pediatric field, and whatever effort existed shows a tendency to decline. These and other reasons have led to the reproach aimed at the Pavlovists by the president of the Academy of Medical Sciences of USSR as we have noted.

A novelty is the recent professed feeding of the newborn with the mother's milk (from another healthy woman) in the first few hours after birth. This is aimed at avoiding excessive loss of weight in the newborn, "Durst Fieber" and also the hypoglycemy which seems frequent in infants during the first several days of life. Another consideration claimed for this method is the transfer of immune bodies. In the West the method followed is offering the newborn an abundant amount of sweetened tea. This method fails to provide immune antibodies but they are compensated for by the tetracyclines and the superior regime and care to which the newborn is subject.

A new method is recommended for treating the umbilicus of the newborn. The base of the cord is dried with sterile gauze or cotton. At the level of the skin it is tightly and cautiously clamped, preferably by means of a curved instrument. Division of the cord is 10-15 cm. farther; then the clamp is removed and tight ligation is done at the groove of the clamping. The cord is cut 4-5 cm. above the site of ligation. Then the rest of the cord is again cleaned in a sterile manner and surrounded with gauze which is well fixed to the cord's base and changed every day. Above the gauze a sterile dressing is applied. It is claimed that in 90% of the newborn the cord falls in the first three to five days.

There is a mania for adherence to the use of phytonsides (the volatile substances) contained in such plants as garlic, onion, etc. This trend was the result of the spirit of originality born of desperate needs and is still maintained. It reminds us of the similar trend of the Nazis in the early thirties. Children sick of scarlet fever and simultaneously suffering from chronic tonsilitis or chronic purulent otitis are subjected to sanation of their pharynxes by exposure to the emanations of garlic! There is a people's wisdom saying, "a grandmother being idle, got a little pig to care for."

Artificial feeding of children was severely denounced until recent years. But some time ago a special committee was appointed and reported on the progress in this field in the West. This time all was very attractive, first, because it enabled women to work and build Communism. Many recommendations were made as well as the construction of a special plant to produce standard foods for artificial feedings. . . . Most recently these artificial foods produced by their industries are strongly recommended.

Droplet enemas are still being used in the treatment

of toxic intestinal disorders and the intravenous instal-
lation so widely used in the U.S. is now being applied
here and there in the USSR.

Transfusions are given also by bone marrow; exchange transfusions in Leningrad were started in 1951
and much later in Moscow. There is no mention in
Soviet pediatric or other literature of rapid digitalization of patients of any age.

Dry cupping is still widely used in the treatment
and prevention of pneumonias, in allergic diseases and
for "bio-stimulating" purposes.

Polypragmasia is a rule. Every child more seriously
ill is given, in a single combination or in additional
injections: camphor oil, caffeine, cardiazol, phenobarbital and bromide, — all motivated by Pavlov's
teaching, and to prevent heart failure . . . camphor oil
is given twice a day. Numerous shots are given to
critically ill children, penicillin alone, six to eight times
in twenty-four hours! This practice is incompatible
with Pavlov's concepts.

The first case of fibroelastosis was described by A. M.
Viherta in 1957! Regarding the nephropathias, they
recognize that "in our country's literature, particularly
in the pediatric field, very few works have been dedicated to this problem." *(Pediatria, #7, 1958.)* Despite
the fact that pediatrics is still a crucial problem in the
USSR and the prophylactic trend of medicine prevailing in general, they do not have the grids as those
worked out by the Boston pediatric group used all
over the U.S. and of such highly practical, instructive
and clinical significance.

The first article on cytomegilic inclusion disease was
published in 1958! "In Russian literature we have
found no indications on the possibility of the develop-

ment of cardio-vascular pathology during the life span of an arachnodactylic case as a result of congenital inferiority of the vascular walls and heart muscle." Thus O. I. Hnunina and A. A. Golovina write with respect to Marfan syndrome in an article published in *Klinicheskaya Meditsina*, #4, 1961. Then the authors describe the first case in USSR. This entity of Marfan, with its cardio-vascular pathology, is an old story in the West and in the U.S. where such cases are confirmed and traced in the parents by finding the syndrome in the children and vice versa. Why has it been missed in USSR? Because its doctors have a little less creative imagination, do not see far enough, and are dulled by political ideology and complexes.

The following case is another illustration of the standard of Soviet pediatrics, Soviet doctors and therefore of Soviet medical science.

An eleven year old girl had acute laryngitis and at 5:15 P.M. was given a first shot of 150,000 U. of pure penicillin (the prescription being 150,000 qid.). At 5:20 (five minutes later,) the child showed sharp weakness, and the aids started looking for the doctor. In the next few minutes the child went into full coma, the skin turning very pale, the nasal-oral triangle cyanotic as well as the tips of the fingers, and the pulse accelerating and weakening. On his arrival the doctor immediately gave a combination of caffeine plus camphor oil, and cardiamin, and inhalations of oxygen and alcohol-ammonium! With respect to the three drugs injected, they were given I.M. or S.C. If any had been given I.V. it would have been pointed out. Caffeine and camphor oil is a Soviet "discovery," surely a fine emulsion. The condition of the child rapidly worsened and at 5:45 she expired, — thirty

minutes after the shot.   Autopsy confirmed that death
was due to anaphylactic shock.

The child's outpatient card showed that in 1957 and
1958 she had had grippe.   Then penicillin had been
given in tablets, 100,000 qid. and for some time she
had been hospitalized with the diagnosis of bronchial
asthma and given three injections of penicillin, each
of 150,000 U.   However, at that time she had not
shown any sensitivity to penicillin.

The account of the accident is not accompanied by
any other remarks except urging care in introducing
penicillin to any allergic patients.   This warning is
given by the Physician (Vrach) O. I. Haritonov of the
Krasnoyarsk regional Forensic medicine office. (*Pediatria*, #9, 1961, p. 78.)

Every doctor or senior medical student in the U.S.
or anywhere else in the world, would characterize
such a way of treating anaphylactic shock, from beginning to end, as one of total ignorance and irresponsibility.   This ignorance, it seems, is also not alien to
the editors of the journal, academicians, who have not
supplemented the article with any notes.   We may
admit that the doctor may have been a Communist.

A great number of pediatric books are published
annually, as well as monographs and articles.   The
best work on Pediatrics in the USSR (600 pages,
ordinary format,) belongs to the late Leningrad Professor M.C. Maslov.   This is a textbook on *Children's
Diseases*.   It first appeared in 1940, the second time
in 1945 and the last in 1957.   It is a compilation, but
of such a wide and honest use of foreign, Western
authors and citations of their original names, that it is
unique in Soviet experience.   The work also gives the
very strong impression that it is written by a gifted

clinician of broadest erudition. However, it is greatly reminiscent of Professor Robert Debré's *Pathologie Infantile*, though condensed.

While the American doctors and pediatricians have a number of pediatric textbooks, the W. Nelson's exceeding all that the Russians have written or dreamed of, the most popular book of pediatrics in the USSR is that of Koltipin-Langovoi and Vlassov (518 pages, ordinary size). It is used as the main book for the training of Soviet medical students, but mostly to serve the pediatrician and the doctor in general. This is so because it is much more practical than M. C. Maslov's, mentioned above. The book in question underwent its tenth edition in 1959. However, as the Russians pointed out, this edition contains numerous defects. In *Pediatria*, Moscow, #10, 1959, an echo was published. Following are some of the defects.

Antitoxin is called antibody. Regarding Rickets, no mention is made of alkaline phosphatase. In the section on Vitamin D, it is said that 250 units are contained per kg. weight, but of what is not explained. Leukemia is wrongly classified (20,000 WBC are said to be characteristic of the aleucemic leukemia). Nothing is mentioned regarding the contemporary hormonal and antimetabolic treatment of leukemias. The diagnostic significance of the CSF in poliomyelitis is not pointed out. The dosage of insulin is given as one unit to two grams of sugar in the urine instead of 5-6 grams. The antibiotic section is full of mistakes.

It is certain to every student in the third class of the medical school that Farina Sinapis discharges its active constituents when mixed with cold but not with hot water. The respectable authors are recommending the latter manner; etc., etc.

In 1958, a new Textbook of Children's Diseases appeared. Its authors are Professors V. A. Vlassov, N. I. Ossinovsky, K. F. Popov, and A. I. Titova. A review of the book is given in the April issue, 1961, of *Pediatria*. However, the reviewers, The Collective of Physicians at the Institute of Children's Diseases in Omsk, find the following inconsistencies (we give a few only): Pathogenesis of Scarlet Fever unclear. Isolation of Scarlet Fever patients for two weeks. Vaccination against pertussis has not received wide recognition! Epidemic parotitis isolation 21 days. Epidemic parotitis contacts, isolation 25 days! Complications from vaccination against small pox are not described. Treatment of chronic forms of dysentery are not given.

Another book of Pediatrics appeared in 1960 by three pediatricians of greatest renown in USSR — Professors, Academicians, V. I. Molchanov, U. F. Dombrovskaya (a lady,) and D. D. Lebedev: *Propedeutics of the Diseases of Childhood*, 314 pages . . . Nevertheless two docents, L. G. Kvassnaya and V. K. Mironovich (Voproci Materinstva I Detstva, *Problems of Motherhood and Childhood*, a monthly journal, circulation 5,750, #11, 1961,) reviewed it and pointed out a number of defects, which we are avoiding here citing.

If the goal of Soviet medicine is prevention of disease, this is mostly true of Soviet pediatrics. There are a great many popular works dedicated to the subject of care for children and especially for infants. All were recently reviewed by C. L. Polchanova. (*Pediatria*, #2, 1962.) She enumerates many "annoying mistakes" in this popular literature. We will cite only some of these "mistakes" which depict the scientific and clinical image of the Soviet doctor.

1. With respect to infants, non-breast feeding "makes them" slower to sit up than the breast fed. So with standing and walking; psychic development also lags. (Author from Kishinev, edition of book, 1957.)

2. The mother breast feeding her baby "should eat one and one-half times as much food."

3. Artificial feeding should be started "with small amounts and increased gradually for four days."

4. With respect to the language used by some authors, I. N. Ussov says, "Total caloric value of food for the infant suffering from diathesis exudativa, especially of its doughey form (French — pateux, in Russian given by the author as 'pastose') should be, for example, ten percent less than the average for the same age of healthy children."

A survey of the physical development of children between three and five for the last 80 years shows considerable increase in the percentages, — height, 11%, weight, 35%.

Deaths from acute digestive disorders and from pneumonias are reduced almost to zero. (A. F. Toor.)

Mortality and morbidity in conjunction with medical genetics, and the latter per se, are highly intriguing Soviet specialists.

Commenting on the report of the president of the AMS of USSR whom we mentioned many times, N. N. Zhukov-Vereznikov says:

"The simplest primary foundations of the mechanism of hereditary transmission have been discovered. . . . Problems lie so that following the victories of Soviet scientists in the fields of physicomathematical sciences, a victory is expected on this front . . . , because a disorder of the elementary genetic activity lies at the root of many diseases more often than we are willing to admit." *(Herald of the AMS of USSR, Sept., 1961.)*

It was pointed out that the number of floras, especially those of the staphylococcal type non-sensitive to antibiotics rises; that laboratory tests of bacterial sensitivity to antibiotics do not correspond to the clinical responsiveness of the same bacteria; that the negative characters of the antibiotics are confined to: allergy, toxicity and dysbacteriosis (promoting the appearance of new strains including pathogenic); the latter appears not only when antibiotics are applied orally, but also as aerosol, parenterally reduce Vit. C and B compl.; appearance of subf. t-re following injection of penicillin; that the American method of acute rheumatic fever prevention by means of long acting penicillin has proven effective 100% in 70 children *(Plenum of Soviet Pediatricians, June, 1961, Moscow).*

At the XVI plenary cession of the AMS of USSR (Moscow, Jan. 31 - Feb. 6, 1962) prof., academician Toor complained because of the insufficient attention paid by the Academy's Presidium to pediatrics. Academician U.F. Dombrovska supported his grievances and insisted greater care for children's respiratory infections. Academician A.I. Nesterov urged steps to be undertaken for an increase of the natural immunity of children as the fundamental factor of prophylaxy against the great number of infectious diseases.

Of course, we should not take the information about Soviet medical and pediatric progress at face value since there is a great difference in the civilization, standard of living and general culture of the countries being compared. For instance, in all of this matter, the doctor means more than anything else. But, as we have pointed out, there is a great difference between the American general practitioner and the Soviet vrach who, besides his inferior training, has a much narrower horizon of acquiring and maintaining sufficient current medical culture, so much so because of the very different conditions of work in which the Soviet vrach is serving. For practicing medicine throughout the Soviet Union is not like in Moscow where all is constructed on the concept of impressive propaganda. Here is an example from one of the largest cities of the USSR. Pediatricians of Smolensk insist that in the diphtheria wards of the hospitals for infectious diseases, bacteriological diagnostic departments for diphtheria should be organized because the pediatricians are encountering diagnostic difficulties.

Regardless of the fact that Soviet pediatric achievement in the purely scientific field is very poor, it is typical of Soviet doctors and, first of all, academicians, to boast and attribute to themselves merits with which they have nothing in common. In pointing out the merits of Professor Molchanov who recently died, it was said that he had the priority in establishing the pathogenetic link between scarlet fever and rheumatic fever, scarlet fever and endocarditis! That he has also "revealed the role of scarlet fever in the formation of vitium cordis." (Editorial, *Problems of Protection of*

Motherhood and Childhood, #5, 1957.) How ridiculous, sad and even shameless!

Quite informing also is the boast linked with the name of the late Professor M. C. Maslov, considered "The Pride of Our Fatherland in Pediatric Science," as it was written on the occasion of his death! He is highly praised because he has established in the Soviet Union the normatives of the electrolyte formulae of children's blood and the treatment of the various electrolyte disorders. With all due respect to this outstanding pediatrician, all this credit belongs to Western specialists, especially to the U.S. clinicians and biochemists such as George Guest in Cincinnati, William Wallace in Cleveland, Robert Winter of Philadelphia and others from whom he has drawn the information.

It is needless to comment much on American pediatric science. We have already mentioned its high standard. It is sufficient here to point out as comparison the electrolyte field as commanded and applied in the U. S. There are only two places in Russia where this most reliable method of fighting children's death rate is applied, — Leningrad, where Maslov worked, and Moscow. But to what extent and how, God only knows. It cannot be compared with the extent to which this therapy is applied in the U.S., and the skill with which American doctors manage it hour by hour at the bed of dying children. Here it will suffice to only mention the merit of Cutter laboratories in this field, the like of which there is no trace in the USSR.

As to American pediatric literature and texts, Waldo Nelson's *Textbook of Pediatrics* and Silver-Kempe-Bruyn's *Handbook of Pediatrics* together enormously excel all that has been written of that nature, not only in the USSR but behind the entire Iron Curtain.

TUBERCULOSIS AND TUBERCULOUS ALLERGY

Tuberculosis deserves separate consideration. Despite the remarkable achievements of Soviet medicine in controlling tuberculosis, this disease still presents a great national problem. Because of this, more studies and writings have been dedicated to tuberculosis in the USSR than to all the rest of the infectious diseases. There are a large number of outstanding scientist-specialists in this field: A. D. Ado, K. P. Berkos, U. F. Dombrovska, N. N. Grinchar, A. I. Kudriavtseva, A. A. Kissel, A. I. Kagramanov, Z. A. Lebedeva, G. S. Kahn, L. M. Model, S. B. Massino, Markuson, V. I. Puzic, B. A. Ravich-Shterbo, G. P. Rubinstein (dead,) N. A. Shmelev, F. B. Schebanov, I. B. Tsimbler, and many, many other university professors and members of the academies. Together with them is the Academy of Medical Sciences of the USSR with its authority, resources, organization, numerous conferences and publications.

It is hard to believe the amount of work that has been done in the realm of tuberculosis. One can count more than 400 articles published during the period of 1956-1958 and dedicated to the complex problem of tuberculosis.

The practical work against tuberculosis — therapeutic and preventive, is tremendous. Professor N. A. Shmelev and S. B. Massino give us the following data, (*Klinicheskaya Meditsina,* #10, 1961): In recent years 50-60 million people have been X-rayed and only in 1960 10-20 million people have been vaccinated with BCG, 4.5 million of them newborn. By government order (1961) the intradermal method became obligatory. During 1960 only, 15 million people were vaccinated or revaccinated, and this is obligatory for all persons up to thirty years of age.

While there used to be great fear of vaccinating persons already having BK infection, now only those who have active tuberculosis are excluded from active immunization, and this is to be determined by a fluorographic X-ray examination not by any titration, ESR, etc. For two decades they have been using dry BCG vaccine for percutanous vaccination.

To the newborn now is recommended a double dose of BCG vaccine. This has been accepted after French authors have proved the higher presence of antibodies and the harmlessness of the larger dose. For mass vaccination with BCG, the original idea came again from the Americans: Spraying the air with vaccine. Of course it is not used in this country because there is no need to.

Soviet phthisiology as well as the whole of the medical science, theory and practice, have their peculiarities originating from the Marx-Lenin philosophy and from Pavlov's teaching. We will try to share some of them with our readers.

L. F. Bilibin pointed out that the first type of reaction of the organism to the microbe is cellular, later humoral and finally nervous. But in tuberculosis the first field to be damaged by the microbe is the nervous system, — its peripheral receptors. Thus in the infectious process, which is, first of all, a process of readjustment of the macroorganism, the receptors are damaged and the adjustability of the organism crippled. The lymph nodes are more involved because there is a primary bacteremia, and the lungs become more often involved and diseased because they present "vast receptive fields" and thus are, more than any other organ, sensitive (reactive) to the infection. In other words the course of tuberculosis is determined by the reactive functional ability of the macroorganism which itself is a function of the status of the nervous system. The nervous system is damaged toxically, and in the later phase of the primary acute tuberculosis morphological changes take place in the efferent and afferent nerves, and earlier in the cells of the peripheral neurons, those of the horns of the spinal cord and of the dorsal nuclei of medula oblongata (in all cases only the sensitive cells of the nerves and nuclei are affected). In the chronic stage of the infection still greater changes occur. (N. E. Yarighin.)

The attacked organism defends by means of non-specific and specific resistance and immunity.

According to Zdrodovsky, in the build up of the specific immunity, there participate the specific infection (BK) and the primary reactivity of the organism, antecedent to the appearance of the allergy. This primary reactivity is the non-specific immunity. The more powerful the reactivity, the less is the success of the infection with BK, to the extent that in fact, infection might not ensue. The role of the reactivity of the nervous system was proved years ago (1951) by the famous experimental model of Ostree: In the lungs of rabbits he introduced a small wax ball loaded with BK. Infection always followed. But when he added to the ball bismuth, infection did not occur. Why not? Because of the induced changes of the lung receptors, whose reactivity had been attenuated and thus no formation of the pathological process followed.

This phenomenon of non-reactivity remains unexplained either by Soviet clinicians or by their immunologist-biochemists. Is this non-reactivity or attenuated reactivity analogous to a very quick adjustment of the macroorganism by means of placing into effect powerful and effective antibodies, or is it a kind of parabiosis or anabiosis of the nervous system? In either case, only a biochemical process may be the underlying mechanism. But while in the first case purely immunological local forces, in the broad sense, are acting, in the second case the nature of the biochemical changes (nervous metabolism) remains obscure. The latter would be consistent with a failure of the infection to take place only if the causative agent perished quickly, thanks to other undetermined factors. But such factors again are inconceivable out of the framework of the immunological (broadly, chemical, adjusting) mechanisms. However, the first thesis, that absolute immunity is analogous to absolute non-reactivity of the organism, that is, non-responsiveness of the nervous system to the bacterial agent, though logical by itself, as far as it is substantiated by examples such as the experimental model of Ostree, is not shared by other phthisiologist-immunologists who find various reasons to tear down the validity of the above experiment. We could not trace the arguments in this respect but even the opinions shared above demonstrate the extent to which Soviet science is interwoven with obscurities and speculative philosophy.

Finally, A. C. Dolin and V. I. Krilov made the important discovery that in tuberculous patients immune conditioned reflexes are formed, and that they arise quickly and are extremely stable. This is debatable, too.

It is worthy of adding here the following with respect to BK as a cause of infectious disease. The course of the tuberculous process is dependent upon specific and non-specific factors, — to the latter belonging, in children, the ready appearance of hypoproteinemia; the immaturity of the brain cortex as a controlling organ; pre-puberty and puberty; the age which contributes to the greater intake of BK; the infectious illnesses of childhood; the more frequent digestive disturbances in children; the more intensive metabolism, etc.

A number of leading scientist-phthisiologists of the USSR like N. M. Grinchar, author of several books on tuberculosis, maintain that the nervous system is the organizer of the pathological process. Other scientist-phthisiologists, physiologists and pathologists object to this. Typical of this is the following opinion of Professor A. D. Semenov *(Problems of Tuberculosis, #7, 1957, p. 28.)*

"The significance of the nervous system in the period of development of the disease, its course and healing, now is not questioned by anybody, but we cannot agree with the claim of some investigators regarding the organizational role of the nervous system in the pathological process. The nervous system appears to be the main axis in the adaptational compensatory mechanisms of the organism." Semenov makes a difference between adaptation and organization.

Such a mechanism is allergy, but what should we think of the nervous system when allergy becomes incompatible with recovery and even with life?

Ravich-Shterbo, author of a remarkable work on tuberculosis, and outstanding because of the originality of his concepts, (unfortunately he died several years ago,) maintained that tuberculous allergy is a separate element from immunity, totally unfavorable and a completely undesirable phenomenon. Other scientist-compatriots of his, share this view. The separateness of the allergy and immunity was long ago accepted in the U.S.

Other groups of USSR scientists support middle-of-the-road concepts. Recently L. M. Model, one of the most prominent phthisiologists and immunologists, wrote that tuberculous allergy in the first phase of the infection is of a defensive, useful nature while in the later stage it is pathological and unfavorable, and is not desirable. This concept of Model differs from his previous one. He maintained before (1959) that tuberculosis allergy in the infected organism of normal reactivity is of an immunobiological nature while allergy in a hyperergic organism is of pathological significance. But what does hyperergic mean in the light of Nervism? Is it separate from BK allergy?

Simultaneously, two other notable phthisiologist-investigators, P. O. Drapkina and T. S. Ghinzburg, on grounds of the capacity of streptomycin to neutralize or reduce the toxic effect of killed BK, conclude that allergy appears to be a phenomenon of defense and not a manifestation of pathologic reaction of the macroorganism which, of course, is governed by the nervous system. This was a smart switch to the shores where there are not contradictions.

The most recent definitions were brought about by Professor P. O. Drapkina (1959) whose experiments have shown that immunity and allergy develop concommitantly, from beginning to end; have the same dynamics; that one antigen is responsible for the arising of both; that there is a link between them both; that there is no decrease of natural, non-specific immunity during the so-called anteallergic phase.

It is natural that scientists, especially in such fields, cannot and even should not be of one opinion. But the truth is that when it is relevant to Western opinions, the Soviets denounce, ridicule and falsify them, declaring them to be unreliable, unscientific and lacking a fundamental and unified basis.

USSR authors attribute greater significance to phagocytosis in tuberculosis than to any other immunological factor. They claim that bacterium of tuberculosis, upon reaching the blood stream, is destroyed by the bacteriophages in 24-48 hours. This, however, the bacteriophages do not always achieve. What does this "not always" mean? It means very, very much because of the following.

1. It is the young age that is very feeble to defend itself against BK, becomes infected most easily and suffers most severely.

2. In the majority of countries 40% of children up to the age of 14 become BK infected.

3. It is accepted that not only the early superinfections are of endogenous origin (most frequent in little children) but superinfections at any age and phase of tuberculosis as well.

4. Over 90% of the population become BK infected up to the age of 60-65. United States and maybe one or two other countries (not any behind the Iron Curtain) are the exception.

The failures of the organism to destroy BK may be attributed to the allergy. But allergy, the majority accepts, is a defensive element, an element of adjustment of the organism. How can it be that it promotes the progress and power of the infection? Besides, in the very beginning, in the first 24-48 hours there cannot be any presence of tuberculous allergy. How can these questions be reconciled with Nervism?

We thus see the extent to which Nervism is a contradictory philosophy on the one hand and how much the role of the bacteriophage is exaggerated on the other. Why? Surely because the "scientists" wish it to be so and because the discoverer of phagocytosis was a Russian scientist. But there is another truth, — the mass of population is guarded against tuberculosis (as it is against any other infection,) not by specific means but mainly by non-specific resistance and immunity. This brings us to the long established fact by R. A. Rich and collaborators, and Raffel in the U.S., that allergy is separate from immunity. Of the same opinion is J. Paraf *(L'Immunité Au Cours de la Tuberculose,* Masson, 1936, Paris.) "Allergy is not the whole of immunity . . . It is an additional influence which adds to the natural and acquired immunity of the patient."

Two other questions with regard to tuberculosis in children deserve special mention:

1. Chronic Tuberculous Intoxication. This is a term first introduced by A. A. Kissel, a prominent pediatrician who worked before and after the October Revolution. At several Soviet Congresses dedicated to tuberculosis the term was discussed with opinions pro and con, but the great prestige of its inventor prevailed and now it is a permanent clinical entity in Soviet phthisiology. It is additionally characterized as Tuberculous Intoxication Grade 1, 2 and 3. Its

symptomatology comprises loss of appetite to full anorexia, arrest of gaining weight or even loss of weight, disturbance of sleep, irritability, overfatigue, subfebrile temperature which is of short duration and recurring or persisting for weeks, arrest of physical development, enlargement of the peripheral lymph nodes, decrease of tissue turgor, more frequent anemia, moderate leucocytosis. These symptoms, — several in number are found concomitantly even in one and the same child. We see that there is nothing original in this clinical picture except what so brilliantly was long ago described by the French authors headed by Marfan, Nebecourt and Debré. Of course the most reliable diagnosis is built on the basis of a positive tuberculin reaction.

2. Tuberculin Reaction and its differentiation from the postvaccinal allergy. Many efforts were made by the Soviet authors to find a reliable way of differentiating the two allergies but no satisfactory way was found despite the self confidence of some that the sea is as deep as to the knees. The majority of Soviet authors agree that postvaccinal allergy, when manifestable should be weak and of short duration. In other words, they consider infectious allergy any protracted positive tuberculin test at an early age. Only in rare cases may postvaccinal allergy be manifested. Such an understanding is considered as having superior prophylactic role by preventing omissions of an early and correct diagnosis.

Further, in non-specific immunity and resistance of the vast masses of population against any infectious disease and especially against tuberculosis the greatest role belongs to the standard of living in which food has the primacy. But here is what O. M. Molchanova, a prominent personality at the Institute of Nutrition, says (1957) on the occasion of the 40th Anniversary: "To this question, nutrition, up to the present time, even the specialists in the realm of childhood, the pediatricians, do not pay sufficient attention." Nutrition is, first of all, a social problem, in the USSR it is a government problem which has not been resolved. (See section on Therapy and Nutrition.) Everybody knows that since 1957 the food production in USSR has worsened rather than improved.

In the field of the therapy and cure of tuberculosis there is also a variety of peculiarities of which we will enumerate some which Soviet phthisiologists believe are of help: long, continuous intake of small doses of bromide or caffeine, by activating the brain cortex, weakens the course of active but mild tuberculosis; antibiotics and modern antibacterial chemicals affect the nuclear substance of the microbe; in cases of caseification, early resection is applied to prevent cavitation; in cases of cavities and repeated hemorrhages from the lungs, division of isolated lobular bronchus is practiced, leading to atelectasis and fibrosis; there is a vast involvement of the nervous system in tuberculosis with no parallelism between the functional disturbances, the degree of pathologic change of the nervous system, and the severity of the tuberculous infection. This all is of great significance for the clinics.

To chronic cavernous cases they give very large doses of Isoniazid (20-35 mgs/kg.). They do this in order to overcome the resistance of BK. The grounds for that they took from American and European experience. They combine the Isoniazid with Pyridoxin, 50 mgs.

daily, and in giving both of those drugs for months and years they have not observed any untoward effects. At the same time Soviet phthisiologists use the penetrability of the skin of the tuberculous patients for determining the state of the lungs, that is of the activity of the process. This test is also a Western invention, not Soviet.

In evaluating the state of the inflamatory process of the lungs caused by BK, they differentiate between "infiltrate" which is the territory of the real activity of the agent and "infiltration" which is the collateral reaction attributed to allergic and other factors.

Chemoprophylaxis of tuberculosis. There is no standard method. Recommended (N. A. Shmelev, a prominent phthisiologist) is oral medication (by means of Fthivasid, a product kin to HIN) in a matter of several months to several consecutive years.

There are many textbooks on Tuberculosis in Russian. The most outstanding of them is that of the late G. P. Rubinstein. It is in two volumes, large format, and contains a very great number of excellent X-ray pictures from the personal experience of the author. On the tuberculosis of childhood, the best work is that of Markuson which appeared in the thirties. Markuson is a pediatrician-phthisiologist. Recently there was started the publication of a multi-volume textbook on Tuberculosis. Up to the present only the first volume has appeared. It is a collective work is that of Markuson which appeared in the professors and most of them members of the Academy of Medical Sciences of the USSR: B. L. Einis, and A. I. Strukov (as editors), A. E. Rabukhin, L. M. Model, A. A. Klebanov, N. A. Shmelev and others.

ALLERGY

The student of Soviet medical science as shown in the journals is impressed by the lack of articles and papers dedicated to allergy. In the three years' issues of six Soviet journals (1959-1961), the writer has not found three articles discussing the immensely complicated and important problem of allergy. And it is difficult to find an explanation of this fact which surely does exist and has its background. Otherwise it is widely discussed with respect to cases of fatalities and complications, with all of the characteristic details: anaphylactic shock, Schwartzman-Sanarelli phenomenon, and Arthus phenomenon.

It seems that Soviet authors foster an idiosyncrasy toward allergy. This appears to be just another consequence of Nervism. Allergy is often a wild reaction and process out of hand of the almighty nervous system and so they prefer not to touch it instead of being aggressive and trying to conquer it as American medicine does by developing means and mechanisms against it even though not always successful.

What this attitude of the Soviet authors means in practical terms one can judge by the following fact: About a year ago the writer read in a journal to which he has no access now, that out of about 75 cases of bronchial asthma, the Soviet doctors in care of the cases were able to reveal specific sensitivity to allergens in only three cases! The rest of the sick children were considered as having asthma on the basis of Nervism.

INFECTIOUS DISEASES

The field of infectious diseases is one in which unusual work has been done and still is being done on the part of all factors involved. When one reads the instructions and resolutions with respect to the protection of children from infections, he feels that the medical people are embarked on a kind of crusade against an enemy that has invaded and is devastating their country. The role of the Party here, as a pushing and controlling force, is of great significance. The achievements are remarkable, though infectious diseases still present a great problem. It is a harder task because of the low standard of living, low culture of the masses, primitive civilization in the greater part of the empire, and the lack of modern antibiotics, vaccines in sufficient quantity, quality and variety, and the lack of equipment. What all this means in the overall field of Public Health and even of morals, is seen in the reading of such advertisements as this in the USSR: "For Rent — Single bed, window revealing attractive view, convenient partition from the rest of the room; a calm, small family." Or that there is for rent a portion of hygienic room and the renter can use a kitchen serving four families only.

Besides the pediatricians, there are two other categories of direct fighters against infectious diseases, — the epidemiologists and the infectionists. They are, generally, pediatricians who have specialized particularly in the field of infections, and are heads on the staff of "Health-epidemiological Stations."

The underlying philosophy is that they can attain anything. K. Bikov, the foremost Pavlovist, basing on the experience of World War II, concludes that constitution is of no significance in the appearance of such illnesses as hypertension, ulcer of the stomach and duodenum, tuberculosis, etc. Of the same opinion is

A. L. Miasnidov regarding rheumatic fever. In the
realm of infection the same philosophy prevails —
that unlimited is the degree to which resistance can be
fortified.

Measles are prevented by means of gamma globulin
and much more by the cheaper immune blood serum.
The latter is also used for treatment together with
antibiotics, sulfonamides and other "stimulating" factors such as vitamins. Attempts to reach a solution
of the problem by means of a vaccination have proved
unsuccessful. It is a fact that the U.S. National Institute of Health has solved the problem of vaccination
against measles, as Dr. J. E. Smodel recently announced. At the last International Conference on
Measles the Soviets also showed considerable progress
in obtaining a vaccine in cooperation with Americans.

Diphtheria immunization has been obligatory by
law since 1940. For 1960, it is maintained, that diphtheria lethality in the USSR is considerably lower than
in Turkey, Canada, England and Wales and some
other countries. In some cities like Moscow, Talyn,
Gorky, Leningrad, Riga, Kishinev, Saratov, Rostov
diphtheria lethality does not exist. However — the goal
has been placed before Soviet medics to completely
liquidate diphtheria. In the last five years morbidity
has decreased five times. A mixed vaccine against
Diphtheria and Pertussis is used but it is "not pure
enough, causes many side reactions and is unreliably
standarized" says a recent acknowledgment.

Pertussis. They did not have a vaccine as late as
1957. Recently they have been using one of their own
on a wide scale. As we mentioned above, the mixed
vaccines they use now "need perfection," as their in-

fectionists say. (For other infections see the chapter
on Virusology.) Following is an echo of theirs.

"Indicators of morbidity of pertussis in the USSR
are . . . at present rather high . . . definite successes
in reducing morbidity, thanks to vaccination, are realized in only a few countries.   Countries where the
results of the vaccination on the incidence of morbidity
and lethality in the entire country are found are the
U.S.A. and Canada. . . . At present the immunological
layer amidst the children's population constitutes about
80-90% and in pertussis morbidity (and also diphtheria) there are considerable shifts toward reduction."
In the USSR anti-pertussis vaccination was started in
1955-56 and later, pertussis-diphtheria. *(Pertussis and
Prospects of its Liquidation in the Country,* M. S.
Zaharova, *Herald of the Academy of Medical Sciences
of USSR,* Feb. 1962, p. 77.)

In dysentery — recommended is shortlived treatment
in order to avoid side effects because of the application
of antibiotics.   And together with the etiotropic treatment always the correct outlining of diet and regime
is of great significance; vitaminotherapy, treatment of
concurrent illnesses, also the sanitation of the surrounding conditions . . . (A.F. Bilibin and I. I. Shtetina,
*Treatment of Patients of Acute Dysentery, Herald of
the Academy of Medical Sciences of the USSR,* Feb.
1962, p. 62.)

In cases of colitises, when the bacterial culture is
negative a specific test is practiced (with reliability
up to 85%) of dysenterial hydrolysate of Flexner type
introduced intradermally.

Typhoid fever is rare in the USSR among children.

Rheumatic fever

September 3-7, 1961 in Rome the Tenth International Congress of Rheumatologists took place. The U.S. delegates gave fourteen reports while those of the Soviet Union, twelve men headed by an academician (Professor A. I. Nesterev) gave two reports only. (A. V. Dolgopolova and L. S. Alexeev, "Effect of curative and physical culture upon the course of rheumatic fever in its active phase"; and A. I. Nesterev and V. I. Sachkov, "A new original method of the diagnosis of acute rheumatic fever and other colagenous diseases worked out on the basis of the antigenic structure of serum proteins.") This type of studies has been going on for a long time in the West and the U.S., and there is nothing new in them. They may be "original" for the academicians behind the Iron Curtain. There is a people's wisdom ridiculing those who unjustifiably boast: it says — "My dear, where you are going to, I am coming back from." This expresses the relationship of American medicine to the Soviet academicians.

As to the differentiation of rheumatoid arthritis they use the same tests and terminology designed in the capitalistic world (Latex fixation test, Bentonite test).

They claim to have a plan for preventing Acute Rheumatic Fever, but what it is we could not find out. However, the American method (doubted by the Russians,) of Doctors R. Wedgwood, C. Rammelkamp and associates, of monthly injections of Bicillin, as we mention elsewhere, was recently accepted as "reliable." There is no question that their plan will, as elsewhere shown, be related to something of the American sort.

In the field of infection, the Soviet trend is best shown by one of the most sympathetic figures in Russia in pre and post Revolution medicine, viz., A. A. Kissel. He was a pediatrician who served over twenty-five years after the October Revolution. He was one of the most respected by the Soviet Government, because he was an extreme idealist and a noble doctor. To illustrate his idealistic and patriotic personality we present a few of his convictions.

1. Our goal must be the healthy child, not the practically healthy child.

2. Clearly all our efforts should be directed to the prevention of the disease mainly — not at the bacillus but at the man.

3. We must concentrate our efforts mainly on healing all bad conditions of our life.

4. The horizons of preventive medicine are, in the fullest sense, limitless.

5. Our scientific research should be elucidated by theoretical premises.

6. Every patient must be treated (continuously) by one and the same doctor.

7. The sick child dies not from any disease per se, but from the complications which add to that disease.

8. Many outer conditions, professional and natural, induce changes of their own in the course of the disease.

9. I always aim to direct every thought of my listeners to the happy perspectives of the prophylactics.

10. Our country builds an entirely new life. Where in the world is such great attention given to children?

There are at every polyclinic rheumatologic offices where children and adults suspicious of rheumatic fever, and any other form of rheumatic diseases, or are known to have such are controlled, followed-up and cared for according to the course of their health.

Children having had rheumatic fever and showing tonsillitis or grippe prophylactically get penicillin orally or I.M. in the pre-school age — 100,000 U. and in school age, — 300,000-400,000 U. and simultaneously anti-rheumatic therapy, — aspirin 0.50-1.0 or pyramidon 0.05-0.10 or butadion the same dose per 24 hours.

As to the goal of liquidation and reduction of infectious diseases in the USSR, this is the situation of the research going on now.

1. On the problem of immunity and immunogenesis, P. F. Zdrodovsky and co-workers are investigating.

2. On the mechanism of transmission of infection, L. V. Gromashevsky and his collaborators are working.

3. On the problem of bacteriological diagnosis, new methods are proposed, such as: test of titre of the phage, luminescent analysis in diagnosis of diphtheria, infectious hepatitis, intestinal infections, et al.

Great pride is taken in the fact of the Soviet discovery and establishment in medical science twenty years ago of the nidus infections by E. N. Pavlovsky, and of the World Health Organization authorization in 1959 the Soviet Union to conduct the First Course on Nidus Infections of Man (five weeks altogether, conducted some time ago). These nidus infections are: tularemia, seasonal encephalitises, leishmanosis, leptospirosis, toxoplasmosis, and others.

Textbooks on infectious diseases have been scanty. Conversely, there are many monographs, for instance, on pertussis, meningococcal meningitis, measles, scarlet fever, etc. Only recently a few new ones appeared.

The most popular textbook on infectious diseases, but at the same time the second oldest, is that of Danilevich. Interesting comments were made in conjunction with the new book on Infectious Diseases by Professor S. D. Nossov. (*Pediatria*, #5, 1958, p. 80.) Professor Nossov is one of the eminent Soviet infectionists and the author of the book in question. The latter is to serve the students of the medical institutions (Medical schools). Commentators were the staff members of the Cathedra of Infectious Diseases at the Second Moscow Institute of Medicine in honor of N. I. Pirogov. These comments give an idea of the standard of at least some of the Russian academicians. Following are some of the echoes.

"One of the most important defects of the book is that the author has paid very little attention to the classification of the clinical forms of the various infectious diseases."

"The most frequently found forms of the diseases are not described. For instance, the severest form of measles is described in detail even though it is met rarely in recent years, while the clinics of the light and moderate forms are not brought about."

"In a series of sections the peculiarities in the courses of the various infectious diseases in the early age of childhood, (grippe, infectious hepatitis, etc.,) are not given. The angina of Plaut-Vincent is described in the phase of well formed ulcerations, but not in the phases preceding them. Little space is given to infectious mononeucleosis."

"Describing the clinical forms of diphtheria of the nose, the author does not mention the erosive form, though it is observed quite frequently. In the section on its treatment, nothing is said regarding the dose of strychnine and the mode of use. The basis for discharge is not pointed out for the different forms of diphtheria and what are the leading criteria in it."

"Passive immunization is recommended but is it worth recommending anti-diphtherial serum! It is completely inconceivable why S. D. Nossov justifies the tactics of those clinicians who recommend treatment with penicillin only for those scarlet fever patients who cannot be hospitalized."

"In the treatment of cerebrospinal meningitis, 'large doses' of penicillin are recommended for subarachnoidal insertion."

"It is hard to accept such untrue claims as that paralysis in polio usually spreads to both sides of the body with predominance at the proximal portions of the extremities."

Infection, immunity and allergy present the field in which dialecticomaterialistic imagination of the Soviet scientists is wandering free from any restraint. The fundamental concept accepted as maxima throughout is the primary role of the reactivity of the macroorganism in health and in disease. The reactivity is determined first of all by the nervous system. That is the philosophy of Nervism. It is claimed that such an example is toxic diphtheria.

"Investigators abroad have been looking for an explanation of this (toxic diphtheria), and have attributed it mainly to the causative agent. . . . The representatives of Soviet medicine have found them to be erroneous. . . . Standing on the positions of Pavlov, Botkin and Sechenov, they have come to the conclusion that the leading role in the formation of toxic diphtheria belongs to the macroorganism," writes Titova *(Pediatria* #2, 1958,) for "toxic forms develop in an organism which in the time of infection, is in a hyper-allergic state, created by specific or non-specific allergens." It is claimed this view is substantiated by pathologoanatomical findings.

The following is the last publication in this field: *Treatment of the Infectious Diseases With Antibiotics and Hormones* — a collective work under the editorship of a member of the AMS of the USSR, Professor G. P. Roodnev, a foremost infectionist. (Published by the Central Institute for Perfection [Post-Graduate-Training], 318 pages, 4,500 copies, price 1 new rouble and 10 kopeyek, 1960.)

VIROLOGY (VIRUSOLOGY)

Following the discovery of D. I. Ivanovsky (1892) that tobacco mosaic disease was caused by a virus, very little has been added by his boastful successors. Before us is *The Teaching of Viruses* by L. A. Zilber, an author of non-Russian descent, published in Moscow in 1956. We may consider it a capital work on general virology. Its author had the honesty to point out the bibliography. Of the sources he used, 1025 were of Western, mostly American, origin, and only 470 were Russian. The latter, for the most part, present periodical publications and only a few books on viruses, microbiology or botanics. The achievements of Soviet scientists working in this field are poor. They have no remarkable contributions of significance for . mankind as a whole. They have no share whatever in the establishment of modern viral clinical entities, such as cat scratch fever, cytomegalic inclusion disease, herpangina and pleurodinia caused by the Coxsackie A and B virus, respectively. The same is the case with polio, clinically and prophylactically. In the realm of the latter, as poliomyelitis was increasing in the USSR, they are using the American (Sabin) vaccine.

They are using American ideas mostly, but following their deceitful nature, they attribute them to themselves. Fresh is the case with the new type of polio immunization by means of the attenuated polio strain virus. The famous and widely known American scientist, Dr. A. Sabin, from Cincinnati, supplied them. The strain was received by Anatoli Smorodintsev, Director of the Leningrad Institute of Virology. This man "forgot" to recognize the merit of Dr. Sabin and was denounced before the whole world for "grabbing credit." Dr. Sabin developed live virus polio strain for immunization, and when published in *Izvestia* it was reported that there were far better results from it than from other vaccines. It was true because Smorodintsev tried it on more than two million Russians. But there was no mention made of

Dr. Sabin's possession of the original strain which he gave Smorodintsev for mass trial. It was just recently announced in the Press that USSR is selling Sabin polio vaccine in millions of doses to Asian and African nations, of course termed as "Russian."

It would be unjust not to mention the living doyen (dean) of present Soviet science of virology, Professor M. Choumakov, now in his sixties, discoverer of the virus of the Far East encephalitis and of the viral agents of some hemorrhagic fevers of little epidemiological and clinical significance. However, while his purely scientific contributions are of limited number, his organizational merits are definitely felt throughout the Soviet Union. The writer had the opportunity of meeting him in Sofia, Bulgaria, in 1952. At that time he was heading the "Soviet Scientific-Cultural Delegation." He impressed all of us in a most favorable manner, first of all by his honesty, humility and valiancy. For instance, he was asked to share his opinion regarding the findings of G. Boshian, a Soviet semi-microbiologist who claimed that every pathogenic microbe has its viral form which is non-virulent; that he had found those viral forms in a number of the most frequently met, pathogenic microbes. Professor Choumakov ridiculed Boshian's claims in very "picturesque" language. The reaction to this was a loud laugh because the honest professor denounced a theory and "research" which was highly praised by the Party. (Elsewhere we mention the characterization he gave of Boshian's claim.)

Professor Choumakov was noteworthy in another respect, — by his appearance. Our attention was continuously drawn to his suit, shirt, necktie and shoes.

They were all, but especially the shoes, so ugly and worn out! The doctors punched each other, calling attention to this, so that nobody would miss seeing the broken-down shoes of this representative of the "paradise" of man. Of course, we, the doctor-hosts, at the same time felt truly sorry for this man and for other Soviet scientists who, despite the dubious reality, were compelled to work and even go abroad and praise the regime that had placed them in such a controversial and down-graded state.

With respect to the Communist dialectic theories, virus infection and the teaching of Nervism, there is much debate going on in USSR which recently showed a sharp switching to conceptions which are opposite to those maintained earlier. In this respect, notable are the most recent statements of Professor L. A. Zilber, the outstanding virusologist in the USSR whom we mentioned before. At the meeting of the Division of Hygiene, Microbiology and Epidemiology at the Academy of Medical Sciences of USSR, Zilber presented a report on *The Evolution of the Conception of Infection and the New Tasks of Virusology and Epidemiology.* (*Herald of the AMS of the USSR,* #10, 1961, pp. 52-56.) In this report he made remarkable deviations from Nervism (Pavlovism). Because of the exclusive significance of the problem we take the liberty of referring to this important subject once again.

Naturally, according to the Soviet scientific methodology, the outstanding virusologist, after daring to make such a great denunciation of Nervism, that is, of Pavlov as interpreted by the coryphaei, had no other choice for saving himself but to resort to the newest findings in the hereditary changes of the serological types of the microbes. So, through the DNA he claims that "the infectious process may be caused by an agent which is not itself an organism . . . but a grouping of comparatively few molecules. . . . Thus to the fore comes a new term, 'Molecular Infection.' . . . He goes on further to say, "the question arises, are not some of the diseases of metabolism linked with a 'lesion' of the tissues induced by viruses?"

By all this one of Zilber's intentions is to prove that somehow, somewhere, sometime the infection in some form survives and justifies the opinion of Speransky-Davidovsky. And he concludes, "Unconceivable is the apathy of our microbiologists, virusologists, epidemiologists and infectionists toward these new facts which have changed our views regarding infection and which allowed biological processes to be studied upon the molecular level."

While Soviet academicians end so catastrophically their philosophical speculations, the question arises, where do they stand in practical virusology?

Grippe and infectious hepatitis with their prophylactics and treatment remain the principal unresolved problems of the Soviet virusologists. Several million people have been subjected to studies of various grippal vaccines. But, says Blohin, President of the AMS of the USSR (1961):

"Regardless of the great work done by several scientific collectives in the course of a series of years, substantial results in the prophylactics of the Grippe have not been achieved. . . . At this moment there are on the way some successes in the direction of . . . two new antibiotics proving to be effective against the grippal virus in laboratory conditions . . ."

Which these antibiotics are is not mentioned. When one reads the story of Penicillin, Streptomycin, corticosteroids, and the vaccines against polio, he wonders how it is possible for academicians to claim as great, finished facts investigations showing some effect in vitro. How naive the academician appears or how vain because, failing to demonstrate something really significant, he goes on saying this:

"With respect to Infectious Hepatitis . . . a comparative study has been carried on between the hepatitises of men and animals . . . For the diagnostics of hepatitis, new laboratory tests and methods have been offered . . . A new scheme is proposed for the treatment of infectious hepatitis with corticosteroids. (In the U.S. this treatment has been practiced since a long time — Note of G. T.) . . . Specific Gamma Globulin has been proposed for the treatment of infectious hepatitis, which (Gamma-Globulin) is at present in the stage of approbation." (N. N. Blohin, President of the AMS of USSR, speech on the occasion of the XXII Party Congress, *Herald of AMS of USSR,* #9, Sept., 1961.)

M. M. Sheinbegas (1961) maintains that infectious hepatitis is spread by oral-intestinal and by air-droplet route, the latter being of shorter duration while through the former a huge amount of virus is transmitted. I. L. Bogdanov (1962) is of the opinion that infectious hepatitis is a purely air droplet borne disease. The same author (I. L. Bogdanov) further writes:

"However, in our literature these differentiations (between Infectious Hepatitis and Homologous Hepatitis) very often are not taken into account. Regrettably, even in the *Instruction Regarding the Combat Against Epidemic Hepatitis* (Botkin's Disease) published in 1958, and edited by the Institute of Virusology at the Academy of Medical Sciences of the USSR, it is not pointed out that two different types of causative agent exist. More than that, in this instruction it is said that infection with the virus of the disease of Botkin (Infectious Hepatitis) occurs by enteral and parenteral route with this difference, that in the former route infection takes place in shorter time, and in the latter in a longer time, from two to six months or more! *(Herald of the Academy of Medical Sciences of the USSR,* Feb., 1962, p. 323.)

In a just published article *(Journal of Neurology and Psychiatry honoring the name of S. S. Korssakov,* March, 1962) the Leningrad Professor A. G. Panov writes on the Tick Borne Encephalitises and maintains that they are induced not only by tick bites but possibly by other insects such as fleas, some mosquitoes and even by means of use of goat's milk on which virus carrier ticks have fed.

Commenting further on the protection from this disease, Professor Panov says:

"Main method of treatment of these encephalitises remains the specific serotherapy although its effectiveness is still controversial." (This serum is a Soviet product, G. T. Note.) And he goes on: "Prophylactically the effectiveness of the brain vaccine has been verified for many years by application to hundreds of thousands of people.

However, well known are also many defects . . .
In recent years morbidity among the vaccinated
became frequent . . . cases also were observed of
post vaccinal encephalomyelitis . . . the clinical
peculiarities of the latter do not rule out the
possibility of vaccinal infection." (Ib. p. 321)

Soviet authors claim that they have produced and
used a mump vaccine which they have not shown to
the world. While this is so, and they recognize that
their efforts in discovering an anti-flu vaccine have been
unsuccessful, here in the U.S. have been in use a
number of flu vaccines — parenteral and even oral
(Oravax-Merrell and others). Simultaneously a new
vaccine against the common cold — a virus infection
was just placed into production in the U.S. A hepatitis
vaccine and another for measles are pending also.

It is obvious that the achievements of the Soviet
academicians and scientists in the virus field as every
other medical field are humble. This does not prevent
them from boasting of great results.

"In our country we have made," they say, "the
greatest discoveries which have received world
recognition:
1. Discovery of the existence of nidus infectious diseases;
2. Teaching about the mechanisms of confer-
ring of infection;
3. Discovery of the virus of the Far East
Encephalitis;
4. Investigations concerning the changeability
of the microorganisms, etc." (V. D. Timakov, Vice
President of the Academy of Medical Sciences of
the USSR — speech before the XV session of the

same Academy, dedicated for the XXII Party Congress. *Herald of the AMS of USSR*, #9, 1962.)

An elementary familiarity with the Nobel Prizes of recent years, and with the history of medicine, shows that these claims are not true.

NEUROLOGY AND PSYCHIATRY

Neuropsychiatry as it is developed and practiced in the Western world and first of all in the U.S. with all of its nuances linked with Freudism in one way or another is violently negated not only by its Soviet counterpart but as well by Russian physiologists, biologists, psychologist-scientists and pedagogists. For all of them, based on Pavlov, Marx and Engels, consider Freudism as an idealistic theory as far as it is not materialistically realistic, "metaphysical, vulgar biologism, and in a number of cases prominent eclecticism" (L. G. Petrov, Leningrad). Another reason for them to hate Freudism is that it had promulgated the entrance of non-medical professionalists into the most sensitive medical field, also of various sorts of social scientists and workers, all of bourgeoise genre, thus still more aggravating the situation of the patient and handicapping the physician. The following illustrates the numerous denunciations in the above Soviet style.

"In neurological and especially in psychiatric science the ideological struggle is quite sharp and tense. Militant reactionary idealism in psychiatry has become really wide-spread in the form of orthodox and modernized Freudism, in the so-called psychosomatic medicine and deeper psychology, closely linked with other idealistic trends

in psychiatry, phenomenalism, existentialism, etc."
(*J. Neurologii and Psychiatrii for the name of
S. S. Korssakov*, #12, 1961 — Leading article.)

"Contemporary bourgeoise scientists persistently
maintain the dogmatic, speculative, pansexual,
infantil-libidosmial theory of Freud. They recognize the decisive role in the life of the individual
as well as of society of sex instincts, instincts of
authority, the invariable instinct of homicide (war)
and so on, and consider most important the
'unconscious and subconscious'." (Ibid.)

The above opinions of the Soviet anti-Freudians are
very kin to those of a number of American scientist-
psychiatrists, among them the late Dr. Coyle Campbell,
a former Freudist and later an ardent "con." He also
is of the conviction that Freud had introduced into the
practices the non-medical professionalists in order to
easier conceal the non-scientific nature of his system
and make out of it almost a blind sect.

Based upon the general knowledge of Soviet medicine which is absolutely dominated by Pavlov's teaching, and Soviet physiology and biology, one can further
see the reasons for the negation of Freudism in that it
is considered by them a pathological theory, a product
of a pathological author. The latter, according to
them, and contrary to even the elementary understanding and feeling of the spirit of evolution, has
degraded and pathologized man. Then Freud and his
disciples claim that Freudism is endeavoring to really
help the same man! This is neither true nor possible,
they say. In this sense O. Herbert Mowrer, famous
researcher of the University of Illinois, criticized the
"moribund body of classical Freudian theory. We

have largely followed," said he, "the Freudian doctrine that human beings become emotionally disturbed, not because of their having done anything palpably wrong, but because they instead lack insight. This leads to the discovery that the patient has been, in effect, too good, that he has within himself impulses, especially those of lust and hostility, which he has not inhibited; we tell him lies in recognizing and expressing these impulses." Thus, "not only have we disavowed the connection between manifest misconduct and psychopathology, we have also very largely abandoned belief in right and wrong, virtue and sin. The idea that man can have the benefits of an already developed social life, without paying for it through restraints and sacrifices, is a 'subversive doctrine'."

This is the spine of Freudism as evidenced by Albert Ellis, a Manhattan psychotherapist who denies any place of sin in psychopathology and insists, "No human being should ever be blamed for anything he does." (*Time Magazine,* September 14, 1959.) Of course, such a conception cannot be a basis for the existence of a sound society and, therefore, of a healthy individual.

Horney points out, (*Neurosis and Human Growth,* New York, 1950) that her theory differs from Freud's in that it recognizes the existence of constructive forces (in man, author's note,) which makes her teaching optimistic, life-strengthening; in Freud's system there are solely destructive and libidinous forces. This is one of the conceptions against Freudism which is accepted not only by the Communists, but by many other scientists, intellectuals and humanitarians. Some of the latter are of the conviction that "the teachings of Freud have been spreading, strengthened by the hysterics themselves with their phantasies and recoveries." Psychosomatic medicine is also severely criticized and is considered "psychoanalytically aggravated." Soviet scientists feel bitter at the attempt of some authors to combine Pavlov's teaching of conditioned reflexes with psychosomatic medicine and Freudian psychoanalysis. "Therefore, overcoming psychoanalysis in medicine appears to be one of the important conditions of progress in the study of psychoneuroses," they say. However, judging by the realities in the U.S. where Freudism is affecting much of psychiatry in dealing with psychoneuroses, we have to recognize that U.S. medicine has suffered a major failure.

Using Pavlov's teaching and methods, Soviet psychoneurologists have contributed valuable knowledge in the field of understanding the oligophrenics and scientifically substantiated methods for training and educating them, though these methods have been known and followed for centuries. Especially remarkable and worthy of mentioning here are their findings that in all cases of the oligophreny, the interaction between the two signal systems is disturbed, the first being the reality, the second the terms, the language. This paved the way to the more correct understanding of the fundamental clinical types of oligophrenics and how to more successfully help them; to the realization that any formation of conditioned links (reflexes) by means of words (ideas) in oligophrenics is extremely difficult; and that the physical performances and continuous repetition appears to be of utmost importance in any method designed to more successfully train the oligophrenics.

L. B. Gakkel, in a published monograph based upon experimental and clinical material of his own, convincingly demonstrated the fundamental pathophysiological mechanism of the syndrome of obsession consisting in pathological inertness of the processes of excitation in separate functional-dynamical areas — "diseased areas" of the cortex of the large hemispheres. In the same manner this author and others are attempting to substantiate every pathological phenomenon of psychiatry by corresponding pathophysiological mechanisms. Neuropathologoanatomists revealed surprising and promising findings in the development of the fetal brain from the very beginning of its life in close relation with the nutrition and the reflectory principle, the latter starting with reflexes from the vestibular apparatus.

In the field of clinical neuropsychiatry and the problems linked with and encountered in the Communist society, neuropsychiatrists follow the classical methods outlined by Pavlov's teaching of sound, normal psychology. However, despite the conditions of oppression, misery and injustice, they, by their different and non-Freudian approaches, have attained more than the American neuropsychiatrists. The difference between the structure of American society and Soviet society cannot be blamed, because Britain and some of the other Western nations have the same industrial civilization and society and again show notable differences from the U.S. In order to support this opinion of ours it will suffice to mention that in the U.S., the neuropsychiatrists are passive regarding the press, television, radio, movies, etc., which underlie much of the psychiatric pathology. Psychiatric prophylaxy does not appeal to them.

What has the Soviet neuropsychiatry *not* achieved? Here are some of the failures and lagging we find pointed out in the *Herald of the Academy of Medical Sciences,* #5, 1956, and in sources of later date.

"Development of histochemistry was paid, up to now, very little attention, which became the reason for lagging in our country's science, in this important discipline, in comparison with the foreign countries."

"This very valuable method (Electrophysiological, — author's note,) is little used by our country's morphologists . . ."

"At the present time, the question of the so-called 'activating system of the brain,' is widely discussed in foreign literature." This is said in such a way as to imply that it has had little attention in the USSR.

"Working out and checking of the data regarding this question as yet has not found sufficient reflection in the works of our country's investigators. In our country's literature there are lacking investigations especially dedicated to the study of the delicate structures and links, and also of the functional significance of the reticular substance within the system of analyzers."

The scientific investigations of the problem of nervous and psychic illnesses are pursued in eight scientific institutions of neurology and psychiatry; also in the Brain Institute, the Institute of Higher Nervous Activity, the Institute of Physiology after the name of I. P. Pavlov, the Clinical Divisions of the Ukrainian and Bielorussian Academy of Sciences and also in 160 cathedras of neuropathology and psychiatry. In the Korssakov Journal (Jan., 1961) we find these acknowledgments.

"It is a question of honor for Soviet science . . . to take a leading position in the world's science. . . . In order to make a break-through in that direction, and not only learn the progressive experience abroad but also to surpass the neurological and psychiatric science of the capitalistic countries, it is necessary to decisively reconstruct our scientific research, taking a new approach to it, with a new style of organization and performance of the scientific work. . . . This means that in the institutions conducting scientific research work there ought, generally, to be used the methods of electrophysiology and electronics. . . . But such research will be successful only if it is based upon reliable clinical grounds."

"In the program of the Party it is said that improvement of the public health service demands intensive construction of new institutions. Here neuropathology and psychiatry are still lagging behind the rest of the branches of Soviet public health."

"We have in mind the construction of psychiatric stations on a loose regime, with 'open' doors, neuropsychiatric sanatoria, day and night stations, psychiatric divisions at the somatic hospitals, psychiatric dispensaries, 'centers of treatment' without beds, etc."

All this is direct and indirect recognition that such research work is not present in the USSR and that the basis has not always been reliable enough.

In the editorial article (eight pages!) of the first issue of the *Journal of Neurology and Psychiatry* honoring the name of S. S. Korssakov (Jan. 1962) we find the following paragraph relevant to the problem of "bringing psychiatric aid nearer to the people." Here the decisive role is played by "psychiatric dispensaries."

"This type of psychiatric aid assures early diagnosis of the starting manifestations of psychoses, their treatment, the social readaptation; creates conditions for prevention of relapses of psychic illnesses, and assures continuation of the maintenance therapy and the prophylactic measures."

In the USSR a pediatric branch of psycho-neurology is shaping up. In 1958 there were 65 offices (cabinets) operating in Moscow alone, and in 1960, 81. At the same time a sanitarium has been opened with 110 beds. The entities comprised are neurasthenia, neuroses, psychopathic behaviour problems and speech disturbances. For pre-school and little children, two homes have been established.

There is no difference in the way psychiatry is practiced in the USSR and in the West. While criticizing capitalistic psychiatry, they copy everything, — the modern tranquilizers, group therapy, etc. They even envy American psychiatry for using hospital psychologists.

There recently appeared *A Textbook on Psychiatry* by O. V. Kerbikov, H. I. Ozheretsky, E. A. Popov and A. B. Snejevsky. The book is designed to serve teachers and students of medical schools. A recension of over six pages (petit) was published by the eminent Bulgarian psychiatrist, N. Shipkovensky. The reviewer is considered an "idealist" throughout the Red Empire, and he is continuously being attacked because of his views. However, he has dared to subject to devastating criticism the point of view of the four Russian scientists. What the crippling and falsifying role of the Party and the regime means here in this scientific field is seen by the following examples pointed out by Shipkovensky.

To the claim of the authors that S. S. Korssakov maintained the "nosological positions" in psychiatry, Shipkovensky objects that this is a pure misrepresentation of Korssakov and by citations of the latter he points out that the conception of the classic author (Korssakov) is exactly the opposite. Then the echoers make a direct blow against the absolutism of Soviet scientists and psychiatrists to explain all in psychiatry with Pavlov's disturbance of the higher nervous activity. Shipkovensky writes:

"In psychiatry, the combined sciences, studying the diseases of the organism and the pathophysiology, presume a fundamental knowledge of physiology. Psychiatry requires knowledge with respect to psychology which cannot be replaced by the physiology of the higher nervous activity. Psychic activity is a function of the brain of reflexive character, and at the same time it reflects the outer world according to the regularities which are realized by means of physiological processes of the higher nervous activity, but it is not confined to them. For the same reasons psychopathology cannot be exhausted by the pathophysiology of the higher nervous activity alone." (J. Neuropathology and Psychiatry, honoring S. S. Korssakov, Moscow, #12, 1959, p. 1507.)

In conjunction with Freudism, A. V. Snejevsky, one of the aforementioned authors writes:

"The selective action of the new means on the physiological basis of the psychological activity of man caused, as the American philosopher Weall says, a crisis in Freudist medicine. Psychoanalysts attempt to prove that the new means affect only the brain but not the psyche of man.

"The shy attitude of some of our physiologists toward the term 'Psychic' or 'Psychical' does not facilitate getting a command of Pavlov's teaching by the foreign progressive doctors.

"For the progress of medicine, the synthesis of psychiatric means has no less significance than the synthesis of the vitamins and the antibiotics." Snejevsky has in view modern "tranquilizers."

The student of Soviet medical literature is also impressed by the attention which is paid to the problem of brain infections. Just recently several such books appeared. H. G. Hodos (Irkutsk), *Infectious and Toxic Diseases of the Nervous System,* 1961, 296 pages. And V. V. Miheev, *Neurorheumatism,* (Moscow,) 1960. Also articles abound on the same theme.

During 1957 and 1958 there were 39 books published in the USSR, popular as well as scientific, devoted to psychiatry. Each book was issued in an edition of from 500 to 3,000 copies, with from 44 to 250 pages at the most. Recently a multi-volume Textbook on Neurology was started. Already the sixth volume is out of print. Its basis is Pavlov's teaching of Nervism.

The newest books on Neuro-Psychiatry: *Problems of Contemporary Neuro-Surgery,* Editor-member of the

AMS of USSR, Professor B. G. Egorov, and Professors G. P. Korniansky and V. M. Ugrewmov. This is a multi-volume work of which the third book appeared recently, and more are to follow. Following the three previous atlases:

The Atlas of the Main Brain of Man and Animals,
The Atlas of the Brain Stem of Man and Animals,
and
The Atlas of the Cytoarchitectonic Structure of the Cortex of the Main Brain of Man,

a fourth one appeared: *The Atlas of Dog's Brain,* by O. S. Adrianov and T. A. Mehring. In it the New Map of the Brain Fields is especially praised as very precise. It is already accepted and used by many physiological laboratories.

Following is a comparative summary of some data in the psychiatric field as is found in the U.S. and in the Soviet Union. (The information regarding the latter is given in the article of A. M. Rappoport published in the March issue of the *J. Neuropathology and Psychiatry* honoring the name of S. S. Korssakov, 1962.)

USSR	U.S.
Specialists — Psychiatrists	
There are no such, but profiled in this field, working in this field only, and "specialized" for some months at the Inst. Perfect. of Doctors (Vrachi). Their number is great.	Have 26 years training — education of very high standard; they number 8,000 plus 3,000 practicing only in this field.
Staffing of Hospitals	
Heavy. Example 3d Psychiatric Hospital, Leningrad: beds, 1550; doctors, 58; nurses, 200; attendants, 600; other assistants, 150.	Understaffed with psychiatrists. The rest of the data is invalid to compare because the higher standard of realities in the U.S.

Number of Patients to 1000 of Population

3-7. These figures are inaccurate for many of the aged psychotics are kept at home out of respect and are not shown in the statistics. The neuroses are many times more which is a product of the low standard of living, and lack of freedom.

Several times more, including illnesses due to aging, the simple emotional reactions—both groups are exhaustively hospitalized.

Readmissions

Their number is very great, which is explainable on grounds of the inferiority of the doctors, undermedication and ineffective medication. Above cited Leningrad Hospital has 700 first, and 4,000 readmissions in one year!

Very small. For the 550,000 beds in the whole country for one year there are about 122,000 first admissions and 58,000 second admissions.

Number of Beds

It is "comparatively small" Rappoport recognizes.

State and private — 550,000.

Type of Treatment

Main drugs: Bromide, Luminal, Chloral Hydrate, fewer modern tranquilizers; emphasis on labor therapy and dispensary and home treatment, group therapy.

Superior because of qualified psychiatric care, superior drugs exclusively modern, labor therapy, tend to shorten hospitalization.

Nurses

Inferior to those of the U.S. — Rappoport recognizes.

"Superior, because they treat the patients more than the doctors of which hospitals are short," Rappoport says!

Attendants

"Inferior" Rappoport recognizes.   Of high qualification.

Hospital Psychologists

No such exist, but there are voices and suggestions they be introduced into the Soviet practice.

Tremendous emphasis upon them, many times outnumbering the psychiatrists.

Prophylaxy

Methodically, organizationally, foreshadowed by the political system.	Insufficient, ineffective, incoordinated, unfavorable social background.

There are 7 psychiatric institutes and 70 cathedras of psychiatry in the USSR.

SURGERY AND NEUROSURGERY

There are two intriguing sections in which the Soviet and the American surgical disciplines have achieved extraordinary success.

On the USSR's part, it was Dr. Vladimir Demikhov, a Moscow surgeon, who, a year ago, announced the successful grafting of a live dog's head to another live dog and it survived for months. This was a remarkable enterprise and, at the same time, a very promising one as far as the "reconciliation" of the two organic tissues are concerned. It is supposed that this experiment was surely an advanced step in a series of preliminary biological studies. Before the scientific world forgot it, the same surgeon announced that in two days he was on the way to grafting a whole leg of a dead person to a girl who had lost her leg. This leg grafting was said to be "only one of many biological marvels on which he was working."

A British surgeon commented on all this by saying that if the Russians actually can perform a leg grafting as described, "it means they are about 100 years ahead in the field of biology."

There was no subsequent announcement that the operation had been done and its outcome. We do not have reason to doubt that. We pointed out this case just to draw the attention of the U.S. surgeons to a pretension of extraordinary nature in a field (biology) in which the Russians are indeed working very hard.

With respect to transplantations, the highest achievement of the American surgeons is that of transplanting a kidney in a non-twin patient, with only temporary success. This attempt is also suggestive of being preceded by corresponding biological studies of tissue "behavior" of which, however, we are unaware.

Next is the newest field, heart surgery. In the U.S., heart surgery started before 1945. The contributions of the Americans regarding the methodology, diagnostics and performances of the various heart operations are well known throughout the scientific world.

In the USSR, heart surgery dates from 1947 when two Moscow surgeons, A. N. Bakulev, recent president of the Academy of Medical Sciences of the USSR, and his first collaborators, E. N. Meshalkin, attempted the first operations. What kind of operations they were, the writer is not certain. But how far they have advanced is evidenced by the appeal of these same surgeons that a British team of heart surgeons come to Moscow and demonstrate their methods in some of the difficult sections of heart pathology. This visit occurred about eighteen months ago.

The above cited authors are the two main teachers of heart surgeons in the USSR. From 1947 to 1956, out of 256 examined, 106 cases were operated. The same year (1956) they published their book on *Congenital Heart Diseases* (412 pages). We will resort to some of the comments of Professor Petrovsky (member correspondent AMS) concerning their book *(Journal of the Academy of Medical Sciences of USSR, #5, 1956).*

"The authors are just briefly referring to such a widely practiced test throughout world literature as the intracardial pressures, but they are not pointing out any figures regarding it."

"To eliminate the right ventricle it is inconceivable how it is possible to open the right heart if blood will be aspirated from the right atrium."

"Unclear also is Figure 187, for the known method of literature differs from that presented by the authors."

"Though the exchange transfusion is mentioned in only one line, a well explained and detailed scheme is given. Unfortunately, the latter is untrue. In it is shown venous blood coming from the vena cava inf. in the left atrium of the recipient from where it is being aspirated into the vein of the donor; in such case the heart of the recipient remains unexcluded from the circulation."

"There are other incorrect statements in the same chapter."

"In Figure 149, the intrathoracic anesthesia of the reflectory zones are illustrated incorrectly and the topographo-anatomical relations of the left vagal nerve and left common carotid artery are incorrectly represented."

"There are some mistakes regarding the history of some facts the authors used."

"In the summarizing table the type of heart diseases the operated patients had is shown and also the outcome of the operations, but the types of operations performed are not given in this section. Many works mentioned in the text lack bibliographic index."

From the above notes of the academicians the reader can form his own judgment as to what are inevitable mistakes in such works, what is accidental and what is something else. In evaluating their achievements Soviet academicians follow the characteristic style. Here is another example.

"The successes of our surgeons in elaborating upon the problems of cardio-vascular surgery are widely known. . . . For the time for which we are accounting, new variants of open heart surgery were worked out with the use of apparatus for artificial circulation, and also a series of surgery of the great vessels, including surgery of aneurismas of the aorta, replacement of vessel defects with plastic prostheses, etc. These methods are in the process of wide elaboration at present in the Institute of Cardio-vascular Surgery, the Institute of Surgery in honor of Vishnevsky; in the clinics of academician A. N. Bakulev; in the institutes of the active members of the Academy of Medical Sciences of USSR; P. A. Kiprianov, B. V. Petrovsky, and also in the clinics headed by Professors E. N. Meshalkin (the most outstanding collaborator of Bakulev, up till recently working with the latter in Moscow and obviously now sent to the Far East — Novosibirks, to carry on personal experience and to teach what they learned from Americans and from the British team, A. N.); of Professor N. M. Amossov in Kiev, Professor B. A. Korolev in Gorky, and in a series of other large cities." (N. N. Blohin, President of the Academy of Medical Sciences of USSR, #9, 1961.)

Up to two years ago heart operations were performed in Moscow and Leningrad only.

In 1953, a method of direct communication between the coronary arteries and mammary arteries was elaborated by V. P. Demihov. This improves the coronary blood supply. The same author transplanted the heart of a mammal animal into the chest of another mammal and the heart continued to live and work, not for long, but it is able to assume the whole work of the "host" animal; he succeeded in reviving the heart in bodies of persons who had been dead one to two hours; they aim before the end of this year, to be able to use hearts for reviving hearts and lungs and for temporary maintaining of circulation of agonizing patients; he hopes that heart transplantation may in the near future appear as the most radical method in the treatment of gravely ill heart patients.

Surgical treatment of the peripheral tuberculous lymph nodes is advocated more and more in the USSR under the simultaneous protection of antibiotics and antibacterials. Thoracic surgery of various cases of tuberculosis as well as of other pulmonary entities including bronchiectasis is also considered in the USSR as a routine procedure. However, such simple entities, as for instance, acute abdominal lymphadenitis, is not met in Soviet surgical practice and in the differential diagnosis. Traumatic diaphragmatic hernia was first described in the USSR in 1952! Another example: not described are the hyperpigmentation spots of the lip mucosa of patients with intestinal polyposis — a fine diagnostic observation.

In the field of Neurosurgery the surgery of aneurisms of the brain is a very actual subject and is widely commented upon and practiced. The Chief neurosurgeon in USSR today is Professor B. G. Egorov, Director of the Institute of Neurosurgery at the Academy of Medical Science of USSR.

Surgical treatment of non-traumatic intracranial hemorrhages, which has been practiced in the U.S. for a long time and of which Cushing was the pioneer, in the USSR it is lagging. The May issue (1961) of the *Journal Neurologii and Psychiatrii* for the name of Korssakov devotes two thirds of its space to brain hemorrhages. This is in conjunction with the anniversary of the death of one of their old great neuropathologists, V. E. Gilliarsky. It is well known that they use electrical current as an anesthetic in brain surgery.

On the treatment of gravely ill surgical patients with anticoagulants, there is an article in *Klinicheskaya Meditsina*, #7, 1961, by Professor I. V. Danilov. This sort of treatment is more and more resorted to.

It is worthwhile to mention another achievement in USSR surgery, and it explains why some American visitors were taken by great surprise in seeing the type of surgical instruments used in performing various, especially lung, operations. This is the field of design of new surgical instruments and apparatus. At the Ministry of Public Health of the USSR, there is the "Scientific Investigatory Institute of Experimental Surgical Apparatus and Instruments." In 1956, its staff numbered 400 highly trained engineers, doctors, physicists, chemists and worker-technicians. The institute is now revising the entire apparatus and instruments used in surgery in the USSR and abroad. Besides, it is continuously devising various new apparatus and instruments and after clinical trial, they are included in the apparatus-instrument "arsenal." Compared to the U.S. pattern we mention later, this institute no doubt is a somewhat bureaucratic organization, because it does not deal, as Americans do, on the very spot of application of the inventions.

In 1960, the XXVII All-Union Congress of Surgeons took place. There were guests from some foreign countries. The Congress was devoted to Endarteritis obliterans — its conservative and surgical treatment.

G. P. Zaitsev (Moscow) reported that the main pathogenesis of the illness is confined to the disfunction of the vegetative nervous system and as consequence of it, a disorder follows of the hormonal function of the sex glands, hypofunction of the thyroid gland and of the suprarenal glands. The long and continuous spasm causes hypertrophy and hyperplasis of the vessel's intima.

He discerns four stages: angiospastic, thrombotic, necrotic and gangrenous. Conservative treatment is indicated in the first two stages. Fundamental treatment is protective inhibition with subsequent conditioned reflex sleep.

The delegates from abroad, mostly from the satellite countries, also participated and the work of the congress shows that extensive research is going on in this field behind the Iron Curtain.

The surgical approach to the illness in its varieties presents a number of different methods: resection of the large vessels with subsequent replacement of the defect with a transplant; permanent deviative shunt and endarterectomy, homoplastics, anastomoses, vessel heteroplastics, intimothrombectomy, use of various artificial prosthesises, spraying the intima surface with Heparin solution in arterisclerotic patients who are undergoing vessel surgery, etc.

I. G. Roufanov reported that during the last 12 years 1170 patients have been treated with the following mixture introduced I.V. in series of 20:

Ascorbic acid .... 5% sol. — 5 cc.
Vitamin B₁ .... 1% sol. — 3 cc.
Niacin .... 1% sol. — 10 cc.
Glucose .... 40% sol. — 15 cc.

Before this method the percentage of the amputations had run 15%; now it has dropped to 5.6%.

A. T. Lidsky and L. A. Zbikovskaya (Sverdlovsk) recommend ganglioblocking means for 15-20 days.

G. N. Zaharov (Saratov) has obtained best results from I.V. of Procaine (Novocaine) but only in the early phases of the disease.

B. M. Mahmutbekov and L. S. Gustirya (Baku) have traced the treatments and the results of 700 patients in the duration of 17 years. The most favorable, long lasting and stable results have been obtained after lumbar sympathectomy and intraarterial instillations after N. N. Elansky of Procaine (Novocain) 1% solution 25-30 cc. with 1% morphine 1 cc.

The newest field in which Soviet surgeons are attempting to achieve impressive results is chest surgery. This is evidenced by the account we find in the December issue of *Vestnik (Herald) of the Academy of Medical Sciences of USSR* (1961).

Chest surgery is No. 30 on the problems list of the Academy. During 1960, the work dedicated to this problem has been carried on along the following experimental — theoretical and clinical lines.

On the general question of "Chest Surgery," introduced is the diagnostics of EKG, phonocardiography, ballistography, sphygmography, pletismography, angiocardiography, angiopneumography, catheterization of the patient in every situation; retrograde aortography; carboximetry; immunobiological methods for diagnosing of rheumatic process; determination of speed of blood current by means of radioactive isotopes; x-ray-kinemotography; spirometry; bronchospirometry; luminscent analysis of onkologic patients; polarographic method of determination of free oxygen in the myocardial and brain tissues; multichannel radiography; cardiotoposcopy; registration of arterial tonus; determination of the total volume of circulating blood by means of radioactive isotopes and others.

On "The Heart and Great Vessels Surgery" numerous methods of operation have been tried and improved or discarded for those which have proved the best. Special mention should be made of the operation performed in case of a second mitral stenosis following a previous operation: by means of instrumental commissurotomy through an approach of two directions (sides); elaboration of technique of operation in multivalve defects of the heart; one moment operation of the mitral-tricuspidal commissurotomy (claim to have been first done in the USSR and nowhere else).

The Problem Commission of Problem #30 (Chest Surgery) and the Institute of Chest Surgery at the Academy of Medical Sciences of USSR have organized the First Surgical Symposium on the Techniques of Mitral commissurotomy. In it have participated 400 delegates including 140 surgeons from 48 cities of USSR (other than Moscow), and the Third Scientific Session of the Institute of Chest Surgery of the

Academy of Medical Science of USSR. Discussions and inferences have been based upon over 3500 commissurotomies performed by the Soviet surgeons. Other problems which have been given widest study from a theoretical, practical and experimental point of view are "The Surgery of the Lungs," and "The Surgery of the Esophagus." Following are the proofs: At the end of January, 1961, The Problem Commission had received the plans of scientific investigations in Chest Surgery from 58 scientific and curative institutions, but recommendations regarding these plans have been sent to 102 institutions. On the basis of the data received, the plan of chest surgery for 1961-1962 was shaped up thus:

1. General question of chest surgery — 82 themes involving 25 institutions.
2. Heart and Great Vessels surgery — 243 themes involving 43 institutions.
3. Lung surgery — 119 themes involving 42 institutions.
4. Esophageal surgery — 41 themes involving 15 institutions.
5. Surgery of the Mediastinum — 7 themes involving 15 institutions.

Of all these problems, the most important and actual themes are determined and top priority given.

Problem No. 30 (Chest Surgery) has ten divisions, each having a committee responsible for its realization. The corresponding committees consist of the most experienced and highest ranking academicians — specialists or practitioner-specialists in each field, from all parts of the USSR.

To avoid repetition we have to point out that this same organizational pattern of scientific work the Academy of Medical Sciences of the USSR follows in all fields of medicine. Under its authority and as bases the Academy has 280 scientific institutions.

Research in scientific work in the U.S. is not organized on the pattern just described. However, the results speak for themselves: the new discoveries in every field come from this country and from the West where the procedure in scientific work has no organizational resemblence to that of the USSR. In the latter, as we many times pointed out, tremendous work is done in every field of science and industry, but if judged by its fruits, it does not warrant the expense. For their planning and check of performance are the most detrimental to real progress in science. This detriment is only slightly compensated for by the team work which is strongly maintained in the USSR, though the instinct for survival and the personality cult do very well impregnate the will and the honesty of even the orthodox Communists thus hampering the progress.

As to surgery in the U.S., we will resort to only two examples which show the grandiosity of the achievements of American chest-heart surgery, which the Russians have not dreamed of during the forty year post Revolution period.

Cleveland, Ohio, now has nine teams of first class surgeons working at nine different hospitals. Since 1956 they have performed over 2,000 open heart operations. Here are the world wide-known, brilliant clinicians and methodologists, Drs. Claude Beck, Jay Ankeney, Frederick Gross, George Clowes, Earl Kay, Melvin Reydman, John Storer and Edward Rambousek.

In the field of essential hypertension, Dr. Harry Goldblatt won global recognition (in the 1930's) through his simple method of obtaining renal hypertension. Twenty years later (1957) Dr. I. Page and associates synthesized the angiotensin and opened the road for the differential diagnosis of renal hypertension and its treatment in correlation with the nervous system and the adrenal glands. In the same field but from its surgical approach, Dr. H. Dustin made his contribution (surgical treatment of renal hypertension).

Houston, Texas. Here we will let a Russian doctor speak. In the March issue, 1962, of *Klinicheskaya Meditsina*, F. G. Uglov shares his impressions of the U.S. which he obtained during his second visit in 1961, on exchange terms. Following the usual Communist method of criticizing the U.S. (regarding segregation and war-mongering) he has had the courage to see the truth concerning American doctors and medicine and to point it out.

"I was once again convinced of their (the Americans' - Author's note) indefatigable labor and amazing effectiveness. With them," he goes on saying, "the drive to progress toward everything new and advanced is greatly developed."

"Two years ago we did not get the impression that American surgeons who do so much are involved in research work. But their laboratories are full of young specialists working on various questions of surgery, and especially on the methodology of surgery of open heart with the apparatus of artificial circulation and perfusion and introducing into the blood of various drugs. The huge experimental and clinical work regarding the perfection of open heart surgery was elucidated in the numerous reports at the 41st annual conference of American surgeons."

"Besides the clinic of Professor De Bakey in Houston, . . . I visited the clinics of other eminent specialists in the U.S.A. . . . in New Orleans, Halverston, Boston, Bethesda (Washington) and San Francisco. . . . Common to all surgical divisions, two procedures are found:

1. The large application of aspiration during operations, and
2. The strictest observance of aseptics."

"The clinic of Professor De Bakey carries on the great work of surgical treatment of patients with diseases of the aorta and its great branches. To this moment (August 1961) in the clinic, more than 4,000 such operations have been performed. In the same clinic, mainly by the team-work of Professor De Bakey and Dr. Cooley, over 1100 open heart operations have been performed."

"Thanks to hard work and the abilities of our fatherland's surgeons," writes Rappoport, "we are reaching the level of the advanced clinics of the U.S.A. in the field of stomach, esophageal and lung surgery, but in the field of the heart surgery, where technical equipment of surgical wards, surgery rooms and laboratories have decisive significance, our achievements appear less impressive."

The visitor ends his tirade, stressing that anywhere you go in the large centers of the U.S., you find similar methods used, thanks to the mutual visits the specialists and the scientists pay each other, and the mutual lecturing and demonstrations.

One may read and follow the successes of these brilliant specialists and technicians. But he has to see them in the process of work, of diagnosing and of reasoning, in ordinary circumstances, in order to understand what humbleness and at the same time what greatness they hide, virtues alien to the mentality of the Soviet academicians. The same high praises are valid for face plastic surgery in America.

There is no need here to comment on the American neurosurgery which actually originated in this country (Cushing) and which is recognized all over the world for its achievements and distinctiveness.

VENEREAL DISEASES

There is no doubt that with respect to the venereal diseases the Soviet infectionists have done tremendous work in order to control the menace. The successes are not only due to the use of penicillin. For instance, in the event of the appearance of one case of venereal disease, tremendous search is carried on to find the source and all possible contacts. To this add the control of the Party and its methodology, to subject to merciless criticism and punishment such crimes as the spread of venereal diseases. This all has resulted in two ambiguous actions.

1. Considerable refraining from "provocative" conduct and from deviations from the official moral standard.
2. Concealment of active cases of gonorrhea and syphilis. Acknowledgement of such infection leads to severe blame, humiliation, and the risk of losing one's job and even residency, by deportation to the deep provintsia.

This all by itself misrepresents the actual condition of Soviet society. Their claims that some of the dispensaries for venereal diseases have not intercepted a single case of syphilis in three years is a mere lie, a deception for the reasons pointed out above. They never give actual, straight figures and statistics but always comparative. There is another very important reason to doubt Soviet boasts. The factor which should be borne in mind is prostitution. This is not found in the Western form where in some countries it is openly practiced and where the prosperity and the unlimited individual freedoms contribute to its spread.

In the USSR, the low standard of living, the closed slavery society and the great dislocation of the populations, youth and adult, by continuous moving from the country into the cities as industrial workers, is an excellent premise for the spread of prostitution. The low standard of living has brought infidelity and hidden prostitution to an unbelievable extent and vulgarization, — the people commit themselves for ten kopeyek (cents). This information is drawn from conversations with visitors of the USSR who have stayed there for months and know Russians well, from some writings, and from the conditions in the so-called "Satellite" countries which virtually, point by point, follow the pattern of the USSR in poverty, hypocrisy, fear and other conditions favoring hidden prostitution.

These realities do not prevent the Russians from violently reacting to any slander. In his book, *Inside Russia Today*, John Gunther relays the story when the "Lancet" wrote that there is endemic syphilis in the USSR. The Minister of Public Health, Madame Kovrigina at that time, said hotly that this was "slanderous fabrication," and she added, "It must be remembered that peaceful co-existence of states with different ways of life . . . does not mean at all that our struggle against bourgeoise ideology should be weakened."

PART IV

PUBLIC HEALTH AND HYGIENE

.

PUBLIC HEALTH AND HYGIENE

Free Health Service

This health service of the Communists is one of the greatest deceptions of our time. For since the medicines are paid for by the patients at very high cost, the government, in fact, realizes profits beyond covering the expenses of the "free service."

The following example is from my personal experience in my native country of Bulgaria, which, ideologically and in merits is second after the USSR in the Communist camp. As a "satellite" this country virtually copies all that is done by the Soviets. We have had numerous opportunities to find out from Soviet sources that everything is the same there. We resort to this experience also because of the actuality of the health service problem of the aged and of the population in general in the U.S.

In 1950, in Sofia, the Bulgarian capital, the First Municipal Hospital was started in the block next to my office and home. I feared that when the hospital opened my private practice in the neighborhood would decline. To my own and my family's surprise, the converse occurred. Not only did I retain my former patients, but I gained many, many new ones from distant areas coming to the hospital to be served. This was because people were terribly dissatisfied with the type of service there: waiting for hours, hasty, careless medical service, doctors changing every day regardless of the pretension that the free health service is based on the principle of having a family doctor; — in fact, a family is served by several doctors as specialists. As a rule people had to wait many hours, sometimes all day, to be served, even for a simple urinalysis! In order to "save" time they go as early as possible to get a place in the front line. At the end, the medicines, very expensive, of local or Soviet production, are often unreliable. The reader can judge by this: an ampule of 10cc. of Distilled Water costs about eighteen cents, American money!

In the course of time (it was as late as 1956) I had as patients children who already had been served by the ambulatory services of the neighboring hospital and who had been brought from there directly to my office. The reason was distrust in the service provided.

Getting a certificate for absence from work is a real nuisance and torment. All is accompanied by commissions, control by the Party, distrust and accusations of sabotage and lying.

Even if one takes the free health services of France, Germany and the other northern countries where the culture is far ahead of the Russian and where the health services are very liberal and complete, they present such a burden to the government budget (so much they are abused) that in fact people are paying much more in taxes than if they had to pay for the private medical service of their own free choice.

Private Practice

In comparison with the people of the "satellites" the people of the USSR have no remembrance of private doctors, so they are crowding the government's free health services, bringing the doctors to unbearable exhaustion. I was the "private" doctor for a number of children of Russian families sent as experts to Bulgaria. For a long time following their arrival they treated me with food and drinks that they were getting from special stores as privileged Communist dignitaries. They knew we lacked such items because all the best that was produced was exported to the USSR. Private practice, though not forbidden in the USSR, practically does not exist because of the low standard of living, the poverty of the doctors and the need for them to work extra time at hospitals and clinics, because of the lack of equipment and the severe housing crisis. Consequently only a few coryphaei swallow the cream of Communist "paradise."

NUMBER OF DOCTORS

There are at present about 400,000 physicians (Vrachi) in the Soviet Union; over 70% of whom are women. It is believed that the Soviet Union is producing annually 23,000 physicians (Vrachi), 2,000 of whom it can export to the underdeveloped countries. In the U.S. there are about 270,000 doctors the annual production amounting to only 7,000 doctors. Simultaneously a great number of foreign physicians come to this country every year. The figures between the U.S. and the USSR are not enough indicative because of the very high preparedness of the U.S. doctors and the much more favorable conditions they are working in. The only serious impact remains in the field of the foreign politics where the Soviets can afford to do with the intelligentsia whatever they like, and to the detriment of the free world.

HOSPITALS

Compared to the American standard of buildings and facilities for carrying on an exemplary, modern hospital work, the Soviet standard is far behind. It will suffice to only mention the lack of closets where the cleaning facilities are kept; kitchens are generally in the basement and thus the emanations spread throughout the entire building; elevators are a rarity and tunnel linking and communication of the hospital buildings are things unknown.

The American hospitals are monumental, extremely practical and at the same time beautiful. There is something extremely grandiose and of exceptional distinctiveness from a cultural, architectural and aesthetical point of view, in sharp contradistinction with the retarded, ugly and hurriedly built Soviet hospitals, that are even lacking in facilities.

Regardless of the fact that the Communists are maniacs on constructing with Bolshevik determination and American speed, as once Lenin urged, the tempo is slow. Here is a citation from Professor A. F. Toor, member of the AMS of the USSR. In it, besides bureaucratism, one gets the impression that envy, hostility and internal battling between the coryphaei are not alien to them. Cries Professor Toor:

"How to explain the ugly, delayed construction of the Institute of Pediatrics? . . . It was said that the construction was tightened but the guilty people were not named. And guilty are, first of all, the 'presidiums' which did not promote, but even, it may be, to some extent hindered the construction of this institute by creating new, smaller institutes." (*Vestnik Academii Meditsinskih Nauk USSR*, # 9, 1961.) Some years ago

"Krokodil" published articles and one cartoon according to which newly constructed buildings have to be propped up in order to pass inspection by the government control commission. Generally, building construction work is so inferior that newly erected buildings have to be repaired from the very beginning and continuously thereafter.

Organizationally, USSR hospitals are based on the so-called normatives. This means, for instance, that a ward of internal diseases has to have in the first shift, to every 10 beds, two attendants, one nurse, and one junior doctor (vrach;) to every four junior doctors there has to be one senior doctor. Hospitals are headed by a Physician-in-Chief. He appoints the entire personnel except the doctors and the other heads of departments (Pharmacist, administrative assistant to the Physician-in-Chief who is carrying on the administrative affairs of the hospital) but are completely subordinated to the Physician-in-Chief. The entire personnel of the hospital is directly responsible and subordinated to the head doctor.

There is only one head nurse for a hospital and she is on duty during the first shift. The larger hospitals have another head nurse for the second shift. There are no nursing supervisors at any time. The nurses report directly to the doctors regarding the condition of any patient.

The OD doctor (The Doctor Officer of the Day) is really busy for everything is reported to him. The doctor's working day is 8 hours but the OD period of time is considered from 8:00 a.m. till 8:00 a.m. the next morning. This duty is carried on only by the junior doctors and the night labor is estimated at a half more than the active hours of service. The majority of the doctors are free of duty after 1 p.m.   Larger hospitals have doctors on duty on the wards all around 24 hours. Senior doctors are frequently on call for consultation, and the time they spend is counted too. These conditions of labor make it possible for very many doctors to work additional hours at various other health services, earn a little more money and thus succeed in meeting the most important personal and family expenses.

Everything at a hospital, — its entire activity, — is planned in advance. The number of operative beds, the number of patients monthly and annually to be admitted, drugs used, economies realized, everything. The planning comprises even the number of patients who would die. At the end of the year the hospital activities are evaluated and calculated on the basis of percentages. And what comes out with respect to the hospital mortality? Those hospitals which show a lesser number of deaths than planned therefore show a lower percentage of fulfillment of the hospital plan! This was absurd and later on was abandoned. In Bulgaria where these Soviet tricks were blindly applied and practiced it led to the shuffling of the Director of the hospital department, Dr. Todor Zahariev, who was ridiculed even, not only for the planning of the deaths but also for the uncritical imitation of the Russians.

From an organizational point of view, the existence of the so-called *Institutes of Emergency Aid* deserve separate attention. They are the best achievement in the realities of Soviet public health. These provide large hospitals possessing wards for patients of every medical specialty with a staff of teams of specialists, working in shifts. At the disposal of these hospitals is a sufficiently large park of ambulances. Emergency cases are admitted only in such hospitals. As soon as the hospital is informed about an emergency case a doctor, a nurse and a driver of an ambulance are immediately sent to the spot. If the case is for emergency treatment and hospitalization, after being given every possible help, he is taken immediately to the hospital. When the patient does not need hospitalization as an emergency case, he is referred to the regional doctor of the "united" general hospital or to the clinic serving the patient's section of the community. This system of emergency hospitals provides tremendous conveniences for the patient in danger because it eliminates the long, fruitless and risky search for a vacant bed at some hospital which might be a smaller institution lacking skilled personnel available throughout the day and night or other means and facilities of life saving significance such as blood for transfusion, laboratories, etc. This achievement of the Soviet socialized medicine is the best of all, together with the climatic stations we have described. The same type of emergency services exist for the neurological and psychiatric patients.

There is another variety of hospital, or rather, sanatorium, which operates at night while the industrial or other worker is off duty but has a chronic illness like tuberculosis, acute rheumatic fever in a phase of remission, asthma, slow reconvalescence from exhaustive diseases. This type of sanatorium is of striking significance for the patients who otherwise have to live in the well known overcrowded houses which are devoid of any modern facilities for observing the necessary prophylaxy. Of course these sanatoriums are not mere hotels but there are medical personnel who provide the patients every control and examination necessary as well as any regime of treatment they need.

Public Hygiene, Air Defense, etc. Regarding the general condition of community and personal hygiene and education in hygiene, there is much for which the Soviets should be praised.

Once or twice a year in every community cleaning campaigns are organized and every family has to clean its house from the attic to the basement and the entire yard as well. Simultaneously commands of citizens are formed who take care of the neglected and dirty sites of the neighborhood, painting (white) the street, trees, sidewalks, etc. These campaigns last for two weeks to one month and involve the entire population. At the end, commisssions are formed to check the fulfillment.

Considering the low culture of most of the population, the towns and cities, as we said, are kept in good shape, — streets are clean, garbage covered and the flies less numerous than might be expected. Visitors in Moscow and other cities and parks of the USSR have been impressed by all the aforementioned features. Violators of the simplest public hygiene are severely deplored by the press and the public on the spot, and fined by the police.

In the schools as well as among the rest of the adult population, all are obligated to get training in emergency medical aid as well as in air and atomic defense. Those who show distinction in learning and practicing are rewarded in the end by means of some kind of public attention. All are given badges or certificates for completed training in the above fields. This process of training and education has been going on continuously since shortly after World War II.

All this is not accidental or the idea of the medical services alone. It is ordered by the Party whose opinion is that ultimately, regardless of the deadliness of modern nuclear weapons, man is the factor who will decide the outcome of a war, with other conditions equal. This opinion of the Party, which is a sound one, is unfortunately unmatched by similar philosphy in the U.S. True, behind the Iron Curtain peace is continuously preached, but always with conditions attached, while the people are under the continuous intensive training to help themselves in case of war "imposed" by the "war-mongers" (the Americans). These tactics and the hypocrisy of the Communists in all they do explain why they do "not" care about civil defense, because they aim to make their enemies complacent while they themselves are preparing night and day for war.

Physical Health in the U.S. and in USSR. Public Health in the USSR is generally reaching higher standards and, within the limits of what Soviet medicine can provide, it will more and more catch up with some of the standards of the U.S. But in many and important respects the Soviet public health now is superior to that of the U.S. This is true regarding physical and possibly mental health of the general population.

Physically the American shows more and more tendency to the heavier figures of body weight. The fat, in unphysiological amount, places more and more its impact upon the health of the nation and is forming already the vicious circle, — heavier bodies, more laziness and slowness, then again heavier bodies. The overweight has debilitating effects upon the spine and the orthostatic unfitness of greater numbers of people, not to speak about the link of cardio-vascular diseases with the overweight on one hand, and the shortened life on the other.

Often linked with body overweight is flatness of the feet, a phenomenon much more frequently found in the U.S. than in the USSR, even though the former enjoy wonderful food in abundant supply, including vitamins. Other causes of this important orthopedic defect are the weak, unused muscles and unhygienic flat, rubber shoes widely used by the youth and uncontrolled by the government as to their harmfulness.

The teeth of the population in the U.S. are in lamentable condition. While in the other European countries it is something unusual and unbelievable to find one single individual who has lost his teeth before the age of 15; in the U.S. it is a frequent finding. Simultaneously the bad teeth affect detrimentally the general health and even more. Their maintenance in a satisfactory condition or replacement with dentures results in tremendous expenses for the people.

Because of the disuse of the legs and the possession of cars which are used even for going the distance of one city block, the bodies of the people are showing distinct degeneration. On the streets, in the journals, in the movies and on TV, one more and more sees bodies which present a sad deviation from the classical shapes of men. Even in the reproductions and portrayals of the human body, as in the advertisements, very often one sees the ugliest and most irresponsible views of degenerated bodies to which people become accustomed and therefore unconcerned and uncritical of themselves. A recent editorial said that in 1980 Americans may not have legs because of disuse!

The allergies which are linked with such a great and important field of man's pathology are more frequent in the U.S. than any doctor can imagine. The writer found in France in one year, among the children of several hundred American families, more cases of allergy than throughout his 20 year medical practice in his country. Much of this is surely due to the kind of foods eaten from early infancy.

Regarding the physical status we find a December 8, 1961, editorial in the *Plain Dealer* under the heading, "Pearl Harbor's Lesson as applied to Us Today," we have an answer:

"The frightful lesson in military unpreparedness which was taught at Pearl Harbor is one the nation will never forget. But what about physical unprepardness for the years ahead — years which look anything but easy? If we have to go to the defense of our country once again, will we have the men who have stamina enough to do it successfully? This is a very real problem and the President is right when he says we are soft as a nation. During the Berlin crisis the U.S. had to call up 755,000 men to get the 195,000 healthy specimens it needed. Of the five of every seven rejected, three were for physical reasons, two for mental disabilities."

"Any time this nation wishes to experience humility," said a spokesman for the Public Health Service, "all it needs to do is to look at its selective service rejections . . . Selective service rejections total about 50%. Physical and mental deficiencies, separately or combined, account for what is a shameful, disturbing and challenging fact of our national life. So serious is the situation that plans are now being made to refer mentally rejected draftees to state health authorities."

"Why should the nation with the highest living standard in the world face the fact that half its young men, in what should be the best years of their lives, are emotionally disturbed and physically flawed. What disturbs the Public Service — and the Military — is that the mental flaws are more serious than the physical. Should this be the product of a culture in which one finds the highest percentage of church-goers in the world, the highest ratio of available medical care, the highest per-capita food consumption on earth?" (Ralph McGill, *Akron Beacon-Journal*, Dec. 8. 1961.)

Physical Culture in School.

April 19-22, 1961, in Moscow, an All Union Scientific-Practical Conference took place dedicated to the physicians' control of curative physical culture. The study of the effect of physical exercises upon the healthy and sick child was given the greatest attention: one-fourth of the 86 reports read were dealing with this theme. The following are the recommendations made at the Conference.

1.   Best physical development is achieved by an all around physical culture but not through early specialization which interferes with the harmonious development of the organism.

2.   As 24% of the children in classes 1-4 and 15% of those in the classes 5-7 in Lwov have shown body defects in performance of physical exercises that have been resorted to, it is recommended that better utilization be made of the school hour for physical training.

3.   It has been established that motion habits

in children develop quicker than the functional
cardio-vascular and respiratory adjustment takes
place. For this reason great graduation should be
observed in the gymnastics of children of school
age. Forcing of children to participate in contests
and in their preparation as trainers should not be
allowed.

4. Systematic sports occupation in childhood
may be considered as one of the active curative
factors, affecting favorably the development of
some of the functions of vision, motion analyzers
(centers) and vestibular analyzer.

5. It has been recommended that it is beneficial for children in the post acute stage of rheumatic fever to be subjected to a training fortifying
the extracardial mechanisms of circulation in order
that they be enabled to earlier start a more active
physical life. Simultaneously dosing of physical
augmentation should follow the data of the pulse
rate and pulse wave during the time of physical
performances.

6. Physical exercises in open air all along the
whole year has been recommended for those climatic zones of the country where such a program
can be based upon sanitary norms. An analysis
of morbidity shows a sharp drop in colds, and all
of the rest of body functions develop faster in
children adhering to physical exercises.

7. Experience with physical exercises for children ailing from non-specific respiratory illnesses
such as asthma, bronchitises, etc. shows that they
are remarkably well affected and the exercises
should be considered as conditio sine qua non.
Similar recommendations are made regarding

chronic upper respiratory infections. (B. M. Matoshin, *Pediatria,* #1, 1962.)

There are twelve institutes of labor hygiene and in them research is going on in nineteen themes concerning adolescent hygiene. Eleven pediatric institutes have twenty-five themes in their plans relevant to child's hygiene.

Children constitute 39% of the population of the USSR. These children for the present "live in conditions of Communist education" (S. M. Grombakh). Many of them are residing in new institutions which were not existing before, such as "united kindergartens," boarding schools, etc.

In the system of the Academy of Medical Sciences, an Institute of Children and Adolescents Hygiene has been created, — "the only one in our country and maybe in the world."

In children's hospitals various activities are programmed to distract children from experiencing of pains and worries regarding the missing of school, of home and friends. This is achieved by means of plays and hand labor and the products are exhibited. Pedagogical work consists in maintaining the school tonus: respect for the elders, planning time well, care for property, discipline, care of child and for others ill and younger.

A complex educational training program is carried on in which the children themselves participate. This is nothing new, but is an American idea as well as in Western Europe, and for a long time practiced in the U.S. and in the West.

Gynecology of girls of school age is also given attention and various investigations are carried out based on history, smears, urinanalysis, etc.

The above information is unveiling very little of the real and continuous crusading for an ad maximum physical betterment of the young generations of the Soviet Union and a comparison with what is going on in the U.S. in this respect, reveals a distressing truth not so much because of the sad realities in the latter, but because of the spirit with which this grave problem is looked upon. Here is how the President of the United States Academy of Pediatrics conceives this grave problem:

"A special program developed by the President's Council on Youth Fitness is being introduced in the nation's schools . . . the current academic year, every school is asked to give a daily minimum of 15 minutes supervised exercises to its pupils.

"We think that in principle this is worthwhile programming. However, we are not impressed with the evidence presented by some physical-fitness enthusiasts who have compared performances of selected exercise tests by youngsters in this country with those in certain European countries. We do not think satisfactory means of comparing the fitness of youngsters in various countries have been developed; nevertheless we think it desirable to encourage more youngsters in this country to participate in physical development programs." (Dr. G. Wheatley, Presidential address for the year 1960-1961, *Pediatrics,* #1, Jan., 1962.)

In this statement besides the academical language and tone typical of every Western highly cultured nation, the President of the Academy of Pediatrics of the U.S. has a very unlively, non-enthusiastic and serene view of such problems whose non-solution, non-clarification and neglect are the material out of which critics and enemies of this nation are capitalizing against it, not to speak of the many other grave disadvantages.

While the President of the Academy is talking to us in such an uninspired and undetermined manner, children are taken to school by busses and dropped off by stopping every 20 meters distance and from there they are taken in cars by their parents so that they do not have to walk another 200 meters and lose their time. Yes, their time, because it is needed for the TV where for hours they will sit, becoming demoralized and melting physically. One can estimate what this school transportation costs; that it is maintained because of lack of classrooms, low teacher salaries, lack of education for a considerable number of the adults and contributing to the deterioration of the health of the young American generation.

Physical Culture for the Adult Population. In the U.S. the physical culture for adults is confined only to bowling, — a game which involves a very limited number of people. From a physiological point of view it is a one sided physical performance which cannot compare with the simplest mountain climbing or any liberal physical game or even with the blessings for the body of some professional labor. The adult population of the U.S. can be generally characterized only in one way: they are observers, ardent watchers of physical culture performances, but not participants themselves.

In the USSR mass physical exercises are strongly encouraged and widely practiced in all offices and plants — for men and women as well. Sports areas correspondingly equipped are available. Mass tourism by foot and carrying heavy loads are also a habitual phenomenon which contributes very much to the physical and psychic endurance. An all-Union contagious example destined to show what the will means in suffering physical and psychic pains was realized by the work of one of the writers of the post war period, Boris Polevoy, entitled *The Story of True Man.* The classical games of sports on a mass scale are very strongly encouraged, supported by the government and the folks involved privileged.

Recently greater and greater stress is given by the Soviet academicians and the Party on investigation about the conditions of health and disease in the far subpolar north of the country. Not long ago the Academy of Medical Science of USSR held a special session on this subject in Murmansk where 35 reports were read and discussed.

The idea which the Soviet government places into the physical fitness of the population is very well calculated. It is that people may be ready to endure physically and mentally in the worst conditions imaginable.

Professional diseases. There is much speculation and discussion going on with respect to the prevention of professional diseases in the new industries. It has been determined what are the maximum permissible concentrations of toxic substances in the atmosphere of the industries concerned. At those levels, no one of these substances or a complex of them should cause in the workers any pathological phenomenon at any length of working time. Even the maximum permissible amount of toxic substances should cause no acute or chronic intoxications. Such are their objective evaluations of their problems and solutions. Thereafter the boasts start.

"The standards we published," A. A. Letavet writes *(Vestnik Academii Meditsinskih Nauk,* #9, 1961) "provoked energetic echoes and objections on the part of foreign authors, especially American . . . because Soviet standards are very strict and . . . the concentrations in the majority of cases are extremely low. . . . In the chlorinated carbohydrates our standards are 25 times lower than the American."

"The reasons for the differences between the Soviet and the American standards" (of intoxication in the industries' atmosphere — Author's Note) writes H. B. Elkins *(Archives Environmental Health,* Jan., 1961, 2nd vol., p. 45) "is: while the Russians have used very sensitive tests of the type of conditioned reflexes, we were relying on the more primitive criteria such as the death of the experimental animals, changes of weight and of the particular organs." (Ibid.)

Then the author (A. A. Letavet) goes on commenting that the Soviet standards of professional toxicity are not based on the conditioned reflexes alone but upon the complex principle of the realization of the differences between the sensitivity of different organisms to one and the same substance and amount of substance, to the evaluation of the combination of the experimental and dynamic observations of the workers' health in the process of their occupation. He points out that at present, standards exist for only 200 substances, that 100 are in the process of determination, but that there are 6,000 substances requiring the toxicity standards determination.

In the U.S. the conservative estimate is that there are more than 12,000 commercial chemicals in the working environment. To this number, at this phase, 500 to 600 are added every year. Of these substances, the toxicological data of only 200 to 300 are known. There is a great lag with respect to the number of products detrimental to health in the conditions of work, in proportion to the magnitude of the possibilities of this country. This clearly shows a neglect.

In the home there are about 15,000 different products consisting of chemical components and of detrimental possibility in one way or another, while on the market there are over 100,000 such products in the U.S.

The writer is not very familiar with the labor field in the U.S. but judging by some facts in the protection of the worker's health in the process of work, this country is not the leader of the world. Smaller and poorer countries, even before World War II, had much superior legislation for the protection of the workers' health than many other richer and more cultured countries. Such was the case, for instance, with Bulgaria where the present workers are crying for the pre-Communist era workers' health service, rights, compensation and protection in the process of labor.

Protection of Motherhood and Childhood. A pregnant mother is released from work for some time before the end of pregnancy but paid and for a longer time after she gives birth to her child. On resuming work, she is allowed to interrupt her work twice a day in order to go home to breast feed the baby. Breast feeding is strongly recommended and encouraged, though it is declining more and more. Formerly the medical authorities insisted upon one year duration of breast feeding; now only six months. If circumstances impose, the mother has the right not to resume working for the period of one year and still retain her job and her pension **rights.**

All this sounds very impressive, but for two conditions. The first is that the salaries are low, — one of the main reasons women in the USSR need to work. On her return from the plant or the office, the mother has to do her home work in most primitive conditions, — for instance, to share the kitchen with several, sometimes many, other families; to wash the clothes by hand; to wait for hours before the stores to supply the family with a pound of some kind of vegetable or fruit. This, not to speak of the numerous obligations to the Party and other political activities, makes the mother doubly a slave, often exhausted to death, but pronounced "emancipated."

The second condition is that all these boasted benefits are very small compared with what, for instance, the Bulgarian mother had prior to Communist slavery. Then she had the right to discontinue working one month before delivery and for three months after; this latter could be prolonged to six months with the salary being paid in full. If any health need existed that required further prolongation, it was obtained upon one doctor's certification and half salary was paid for the second six month period.

The Communists took over and had to apply these bourgeoise laws. It was apparent that they were far superior to the Soviet regulations but this was a real provocation, — an offense to the paradise of the proletariat, - so all was changed to comply with Soviet social legislation. While this was not too disagreeable with respect to motherhood, the male workers were robbed and abused by legislation which was considerably more unfavorable than what they had had under capitalist rule. Even today the workers in Bulgaria lament the loss of that golden time which they failed to value at the time they had it.

What was said regarding the fate of the mother and the father is much more relevant to the children as dependent upon their parents. This is well illustrated by the following example.

In Bulgaria there were and still are Soviet experts coming. They are undoubtedly among the best specialists and are considered privileged at home. They are of every specialty, including Government Security and political instructors. They are accompanied by their families and have, as remuneration, fantastic salaries. At the rate of the Bulgarian national currency of 1947 when a high official, government servant, doctor, engineer or specialist was getting up to 20,000 a month, the Soviet experts were obtaining from 150,-000 to 300,000 or even 400,000. This is not a guess but I myself have heard it personally from the mothers whose children I had to treat.

Those people, on their arrival from the Soviets, had a very poor and ugly appearance, that evoked the laughter of every Bulgarian who hated them. They were talked about in every circle, family and group of friends. But shortly after getting the first huge salary and spending it at the privileged stores, their appearance quickly changed. It must be admitted that the new clothes they were wearing fitted them but were of such taste as a horse saddle would fit and look on the back of a donkey. They again were the object of ridicule wherever they went. Upon leaving the country they would buy anything "interesting" from fur coats for the ladies to majestic leather winter top coats for the men. And on their return to the USSR, all that was confiscated by the border customs officers.

This example gives direct evidence of the standard of living of the Soviet mothers and children in their homeland. With this information the reader can have a more correct understanding of the nature and extent of the government's care for the children. No doubt they are without precedence. This is the impression one obtains whenever he becomes acquainted with what is being done for children of all ages. This is substantiated by details dispersed throughout this paper. But again, American children are far better cared for.

The *Journal of Protection of Motherhood and Childhood* publishes 5,750 copies. These copies are spread throughout the Communist empire, to the West, and even to the U.S. One can judge the number of copies which go to the various libraries and institutions of the USSR and the number which directly reach Soviet doctors. Another discrepancy between boasts and facts!

MENTAL AND MORAL HYGIENE

Much of man's pathology and welfare is linked with moral hygiene. It is therefore obligatory for us to discuss here the role of medical sciences in the attainment of a sound life for man and his society.

Mental and Moral Hygiene in the U.S. Organized moral-mental education is carried by four factors: the family, the Church, the Military and the School. From a classical point of view and in comparison with what is going on in the other Western countries, behind the Iron Curtain and anywhere throughout the world, the influence of the school is inadequate and in many respects decadent. The influence of the military factor is confined to a very limited number of young people comprising a comparatively late age following education, mostly in the high school. It is highly constructive but unfortunately of very short duration in our times of deadly peril and complacency.

We intentionally avoid commenting on the family role which is inadequate. It will suffice to only point out that this great factor of life has little attention in the education of the children.

But the main factor maintaining the moral-mental hygiene should be the Holy Church. In a comparative sense, that which the Party is, behind the Iron Curtain, is the role of the Church in the U.S. It encompasses the man in the U.S. from birth to death and determines almost the entire behaviour, thinking and sense of fulfillment of nearly every American. It has succeeded in doing that, thanks to one main factor, — the failure of the American intelligentsia on the local level; for it contributes very little or nothing to the enlightenment of the people. In this respect the American intelligentsia, and first of all the American doctor, compared to any other in history or to others today, is far behind. And no intelligentsia at any level and site can be compared with the intelligentsia of Russia, old and new, as a fighter for the happiness of people. One wonders what would happen to the American society, were not the Church to carry on such a tremendous moral education work. Unfortunately, the Holy Church is Church. Its possibilities and abilities are limited and far from satisfactory for the present space age and with the ideology of Communism as maintained by lies, attractive slogans, deception and promises. The tremendous number of Communists, Catholic and Protestant, all over the Western world also shows the inadequacy and the failure of the Church ideology.

Thus the state of mental health, in the largest sense of the word, in the U.S. is something that shocks every friend of this great, noble nation and every lover of freedom. It disturbs not only because of the magnitude of its deterioration or because of its concomitance with more religious activity than in the rest of the world. The horrible concern comes mainly from the fact that it is accepted as a hard reality of life against which there is little or no obligatory prophylaxis. It is officially recognized and preached by the professionals in the field of mental health that one out of every three or four Americans is susceptible to mental illness and that children, for healthy mental development, need to know that they are loved, accepted and protected by their parents. These two postulations are subversive of the natural, instinctive powers of man; they undermine his will to be good and healthy and his self-confidence. How many will fail to love their children or be unable to withstand the hardships and conflicts if forty million Americans will become mentally ill at one time or another?

Everybody who is disturbed is referred for professional help to the psychiatrists, doctors, psychologists, sociologists, social workers, social psychologists and guidance centers. Delinquents and criminals in great percentage are committed to the mental hospitals where generally they are found to be irresponsible. Thus many are doomed to permanent psychotic disorders. Others are acquitted of responsibility for the crimes they have committed.

It is a rule, even natural one, that every professionalist will place the aplomb of his specialty, of his field in interpreting the behavior of a certain patient or person. And the truth is that the great number of those professionalists are deliberate or unconscious Freudians of some nuance. They explain that the actions of their patients are a product of inborn drives, of temporary obsession, against which man is powerless.

Sociologists attribute delinquency to the social environment and pronounce innocent every human being. They do not fight the roots of the evil, they "guide" and negotiate with it as two years ago the sociologists did with the New York stabbing gangs and the foremost columnist Raymond Moley characterized the approach as a crime itself. Lack of virtue of any sort is not sufficiently considered a determining factor in human behavior and in selecting the approach to those delinquents, criminals and sociopaths. What this all means one can judge by remembering that Jesus made the miracles by means of the fate of the unfortunate, that is – through their will to be healthy. So he confined everything to them, to the person's will. And we, spoiled by Freudism, saltless Christianity and lack of sufficient responsibility are letting things go as they may, not demanding anything great of any and first of all of ourselves. This all has greater bearing on our survival or failure in the global battle against Communism than we are able to imagine. For Communism is an open foe whom we do know, more or less, but we are unaware that our Freudism, distorted and complacent Christianity, lack of fighting spirit, and even of romanticism so characteristic of Christ and His disciples, are contributing much to the spectacular successes of our deadly enemy.

Judging by Freud's acknowledgements and his "teaching," one draws the definite conclusion that his Jewish nationality "has been a question unsolved for him." Freud grew up in an epoch when anti-Semitism was on the rise and reaching its peak, shattered such brilliant and noble personalities even as Stephan Zweig. This as a revenge led Freud not only to develop an inferiority complex but at the same time a hidden tremendous hatred of mankind as an unreasonable creation. He could not, of course, demonstrate conscientiously and openly his contempt for mankind, neither strike a direct blow. So he used his genius to downgrade man and undermine his very existence by pathologizing him in the framework of the family: the fundamental cell of society and the primary humanizing factor. "The yen to 'psychoanalyze'," Dr. Coyne Campbell a former American Freudist, says, "abnormal feelings, behavior and thinking, seems . . . an abnormality in itself, and psychoanalysis an endeavor to explain the normal aspects of life from the standpoint of the abnormal." Through it is rejected any sense of the goodness of human nature, and therefore of Christianity, morality, faith and belief in human kindness and responsibility.

Regarding the Freudian explanation of man's psychoses, Dr. Coyne Campbell further writes: ". . . the belief that every illness and abnormality is determined by too little or too much love from parents, with a concomitant improper attitude of the parent toward sex, is undoubtedly the most absurd travesty that has befallen mankind."

M. Radzinski writes about Freudism:

"This has not been without detriment to the social structure of America. For example, by pointing the accusing finger at parents as the chief factor in the anti-social behavior of children, by means of their voluminous propaganda they (the Freudists, A.N.) have prevailed upon parents, educators, physicians and lawmakers to follow the permissive (coddling) approach to the headstrong exuberance of youth. They have helped to sow the seeds from which the present generation is reaping the bitter fruits of juvenile delinquency."

So deep is the impact of Freudism, so subversive the conceptions of building up a sound human character and soul, that even annually a mental health week was set on the occasion of which the attention of the whole nation is to be alerted. In fact, this is shocking because of its ruinous effect upon the world prestige of the nation which must be the leader of mankind, which is destined to be a savior of mankind from slavery and misery and which must be spared all this humiliation and pathology if it is to offer other roads to building a healthy individual and society.

Freudism is not science, because it rests upon delusions and suggestions from the analyst to the analyzed, the former being the interpreter of what the patient is "revealing." And so there are as many different interpretations as there are analysts of one and the same "fact" of confession. Science works with definite, precise facts and elements while Freudism is only a general methodological premise, all the rest being a pathological phantasy.

Modern achievements of medicine, the tranquilizers selectively and completely changing the flow of thinking and feeling by the psychotic patient are impressive denouncers of Freudism. This surely is attained by means of primary changes of brain cell metabolism. In other words, psychoses are a result of pathological changes in brain chemistry and not abstractions deriving from pathological drives, experiences and feelings on the part of man from his infancy.

The destructive impact of Freudism over our society and the individual is immense. The danger from it is still greater because it is supported by forces against which the most devoted patriots or scientists can fight only with dubious success. It is time for doctors to arise and stop being victims of a false, anti-human and destructive invention and theory which is endangering the very existence of our free society.

Writes R. McGill (*Akron Beacon Journal, Dec. 8, 1961*) "Dr. Will Menninger, of Kansas, is one of the ablest of our psychiatrists and probably the best known. What he has to say reads almost tritely and yet, he has proved it beyond dispute.

" 'For the best mental health, for the greatest emotional maturity,' he has said, 'the individual should have a cause, a mission, and an aim in life that is constructive and big enough that he has to keep working on it. Good causes with constructive opportunities exist in every community.

" 'There is still,' he insists, 'validity in the old admonition, "If you would save your life, lose it." That is basic to mental good health and following it is an indication of emotional maturity.'

"Whatever the remedy, no nation in which half

its young men of military service age are mentally and physically unfit for service can afford complacency."

A citation only from the director of FBI who bases his judgments on a worldwide information source regarding the nature, the magnitude and the significance of crime and delinquency in the U.S. will suffice to shock every American, every friend of Americans and every one concerned about the fate of our free world and its bulwark: the U.S. It will reveal the immensity of the failure of us all: political and moral leaders, intelligentsia, teachers, Christians.

As the fate of a great number of mentally ill patients, delinquent and criminal people is often decided in the offices of the professionalists, so a still greater number of them derive directly from our TV, Radio, Literature and Press. More than that: in those sources of pathology we find crime not only undeplored and unexposed; we find it inadequately motivated or not motivated at all. From classicism we know what it means for one to commit a crime and what it means to him after he has committed it. Recall ancient classics, Shakespeare, Hugo, Zola, Dostoevsky! The crime we see in the U.S. is unmotivated or insufficiently motivated. It is shown like any man, youth or woman, at any time and site may draw a revolver or dagger and kill anybody without the slightest reasonable grounds. And if there are witnesses, they will run away or remain on the spot without making any move, or showing any sign of distress and sorrow.

We will resort to a humble example which, no doubt, has the most dulling impact upon the soul of American young generations. On one of the channels of TV it was shown that a nice girl of a well-to-do family had invited a friend for dinner at her home — a young man who was very poor but reasonable. It was Sunday and she and her parents were anxiously waiting for the young man to come at the appointed time. Unfortunately the boy met with something as tragic as what Gogol described in his *The Top Coat* concerning which the Russian literary critic Belinsky wrote that the entire guard of Russian classics of the 19th century came out. The boy without any reason was attacked by three teenagers who beat and stabbed him. He was lying on the street in semi-consciousness. At one time a girl of about 7-8 years of age found him dying. He, with the last of his strength asked her to help him to call anyone from the nearby houses — 15 yards distant. The girl refused, each time the young man was beseeching her. Then she ran away! Meanwhile the girl friend, knowing that the boy was a good mannered and honest person and having a premonition after waiting beyond the set time, rushed to the home of the young man and on the way found him dead on the street. The author has ascribed to the girl an inhuman and untrue role, but one which unveils the sort of art offered children.

This story reminds me of another I read years ago. It was written by a Russian lady of the time of the Russian emperors. A girl of about 7 or 8 had the habit of wandering in the forest at some distance from their home. One day, when she had penetrated deep into the woods, suddenly she noticed a man in very poor condition, — exhausted, thin and bearded. He explained to her that he was being hunted by the police because of his ideas against the despotic, anti-people government. He also asked her not to tell anybody; otherwise he would be lost. The girl was at first frightened but later was so moved that she ran to her home and without telling her mother began to take food and water to him daily.

Of course this stand of ours will be violently denied, regardless of the above depicted pathology being of such painful concern for so many brilliant and most conscientious Americans, who are wondering how to find a clue to stop it. That the professionals, — psychiatrists and allies, — have failed is very apparent also from the fact that other industrialized and free countries of superb law and balance like those of northern Europe (Switzerland, Denmark, Holland, Belgium, Sweden, Norway, etc.) do far differently.

Human society is not perfect. It has never been devoid of false trends and drives in science, art, philosophy religion and ideologies. Along with the basic virtue, thanks to which the society is coherent, organized and progressive, phenomena of a very primitive nature may exist and remain unrecognized. Conversely, they may acquire the pretense of possessing higher values and that they are fighting for them. Of such a nature are all of the "isms," including Nazism, Communism and Freudism.

It is true, and such is our opinion, that some of the American pathology appears unavoidable, something like a ransom in order to maintain the basic freedoms and unrivaled prosperity. But as it is, it is too excessive, it is a disgrace and shame incompatible with the vital interests of this country, with Christianity, patriotism and survival.

The redeemer of this unbelievable tragedy is the society which has to support the mental hospitals run in Freudian spirit and consuming up to 36% of the state's budgets, thus presenting an insurmountable handicap. These hospitals are full of people of all ages but mostly between 18 and 40 where they are subjected to a regime of irresponsibility and laziness, to the neglect of obligations and to alienation from their jobs, homes and families. The worst is that their mental condition becomes an accepted, iron hard fact which they would hardly ever be able to hope to overcome, and have only to continue to rely on the professional "help." Few are considered guilty. All this makes American intellectuals cry out their grave concern.

". . . That nation is in danger. . . . It is time to revive the idea that there is such a thing as sin. It is time that we brought self-discipline back into style. Let there be a fresh breeze — of new honesty, new idealism, new integrity." (J. L. Jones, Editor, *Tulsa Tribune, Reader's Digest*, March, 1962, p. 80, *America's Moral Crisis.*)

But revival must come from the leadership in the form of placing before the people new, great ideas. For this nation possesses a virtue in greater amount than any other in the world. It is conformism in a higher form from a biological, moral, political and military point of view. The trust of people in the leaders, the national solidarity, are so superb that complacently people have placed their whole fate in the hands of the leaders not interested in the grave political problems of our epoch. Because of this, if the leadership fails to be on the level required not only for survival but for a victory over the forces of slavery and darkness, the great virtue of conformism pointed out above will serve to the peril of the entire free world.

Consequently we can imagine the tremendous impact of an active involvement of the AMA in a broader legislative program and an intensive educational work relevant to the aspects of mental-moral hygiene of the nation and on the international ideological front. The AMA with its epochal achievements in the field of medical science has contributed immensely to building up the great image of the U.S., and in recent years, to decrease the process of degradation of the same image as the result of Communist propaganda on the one hand and of many and varying mistakes on the part of the Americans themselves on the other hand. And a substantial portion of mistakes are due to the bad manner in which the Americans present their country and culture before the rest of the world. If this is not realized and in time rectified, everything may be lost in our generation. And the ultimate destination of medicine is the survival of life with all of its attributes of freedom, happiness and justice. "Neutrality" (passivity) serves the enemies of humanity. Jesus warned: "He who is not with me is against me."

Moral and Mental Hygiene in USSR. The population of the USSR consists of two main categories: the Party members and those out of the Party which numbers about seven to eight million while the whole country has over two hundred million. The difference between the two is not only one of classes of economical or political background. This is not at all sufficient for the one class to feel unhappy or oppressed. We have societies in the West, in the U.S. also, where there is not at all economic or political equality but the people are very happy and societies stable and coherent. The Russian difference is great and repulsive.

The meanness of the Communists is unmatched. Take for example alcoholism, which is blooming in the

USSR and everywhere behind the iron curtain. There is alcoholism and consumption of much alcohol in the U.S. But while in the latter, people generally drink because they can afford to or for pleasure and without troubles; in the USSR, under Communism, people drink because of desperation. And this is encouraged by the government by every possible means because it makes the masses less pretentious and dangerous. This is done also by the Party to draw huge profits without which the government machinery cannot move along.

There is another element in the Soviet realities which makes their system and society ideologically and morally unstable and weak, viz., that the Party considers that it possesses the right to be the boss of the people, to indoctrinate them, therefore, to subject to control the entire life of every individual and to punish or put to death any one who disagrees. This goes while the same Party is growing into mistakes, deviations from the doctrine and in crimes. The revelations made by Mr. Khrushchev during the 30 year reign of Stalin are nothing in comparison with what really occurred under Communism. Any page of any of the post revolution Soviet writers is a tragedy in the sense that people behind the Iron Curtain have lived, now live, and, therefore, will continue to live under a regime of suppression, of duplicity, of fear, of poverty and of moral degradation.

Man under Communism is nothing. At any time he may be moved, imprisoned, suspected, deported, accused and destroyed. The same has occurred and will occur with whole tribes and populations, like the savage destructions and deportations of the Kulaks, the Caucasus populations, the Jewish people. Today any one of us has the right and the obligation to declare to the Communists that they cannot, as once Lermontov said in his famous poem, with all of their blood, wash out the innocent blood of their victims. Never will historians, writers and poets be able to describe and learn the whole magnitude and horror of which the Communists are the authors, and whom the academicians try to present to the world as its benefactors.

Once, Sir Winston Churchill in Biblical words described the significance of the home, it being a fortress of freedom for a man, but at dawn the NVD agents come, take the father of the family and he disappears forever. More than that, the wife had to be against her husband, brother against brother, neighbor against neighbor and son against father. Like in the middle ages, people have to gather in the dark, speak in low voices, in the basement, with radios and telephones covered.

Simultaneously the Party is preaching the higher principles of morality, freedom, justice and equality though, as Mr. Milovan Djilis proved there are many classes in the Communist "classless" society. The entire history of mankind and of Russia was perverted and falsified in order to serve the goals of the Party. The so-called progressive great men of the 19th century, the second half, are continuously pointed out as predecessors of the Communists and as fighters for society of the Bolshevik type. The names of Chernishevsky, Dobrolubov, Lavrov, Gerzen and many other political and literary geniuses are thousands of times repeated every day, quoted, and used as the basis for destruction and enslavement. But the Soviet citizen and all the youth are very well acquainted with history and those personalities. And the contrast between what they were, and fought for, and what the Communists are, and are presenting, is horrible and can make politically sensitive folks, as Russians are, really mad, distrustful of the regime and unfortunate because of their helplessness to speak the truth and to oppose. Here is an example of the extent to which the Communists may abuse history and may make every one unfortunate.

In 1840, Etienne Cabet published his work, *Voyage en Icarie,* an analogue of Moor's *Utopia.* On reading this book, Nicolai Gerzen, by some considered to be one of the greatest and most noble of Russian intellectuals, exclaimed: "The social order Cabet is visualizing is nothing but a *Brotherhood in Captivity."* Of course this world of Cabet was a real paradise in comparison with the Communist order. This means that Gerzen, had he lived under Communism, would never have approved it, and, therefore, he would have perished. This is clear to every intelligent non-Communist Russian. This does not prevent the Communists from abusing his name thousands of times a day. The reader will never be able to imagine what this all means for man's soul. Only living under Communism, behind the Iron Curtain, will enable one to understand and feel as personal the tragedy of Boris Pasternak or that in the background of *Not By Bread Alone* by Dudintsev. It is not proper for the writer of this study to describe his own case as a proof.

All this, the reality under Communism, is, in fact, a great crime. We pointed out that in the U.S. there is also crime. But it is mostly a result of the enormous freedom of the people. Simultaneously this crime is fought every day by the whole nation, starting with the President and the Constitution itself. In the USSR the crime is organized and maintained by the Party itself, which means by the government and grounded on the constitution! And this crime is hidden from the rest of the world by the Iron Curtain. Otherwise everyone would escape as millions did, because under such a regime there cannot be a healthy moral-mental life and happiness.

And this order which is the greatest anomaly in the history of mankind, — which must make any human-being feel ashamed and dreadful, — which exceeds all that the Nazi inflicted upon the world, — this order the nice Soviet academicians are attempting to sell to us by all kinds of hypocrisy and deceit, — in which they themselves do not believe but work for it because it provides them the privileges and superiority over the poor and the humble. Alas, the evil does not end here. It is greater because many of us, Christians and lovers of freedom, believe them despite the opposite conceptions of our governments. Thus we work directly and indirectly against our own countries, against ourselves, and for the cause of Communism.

VITAL STATISTICS

We will confine our notes to only some bio-social aspects of the subject. It seems that Soviet vital statistics are no less a government secret than the military ones. Only occasionally and in recent years one finds figures from which definite conclusions can be drawn.

For instance, it is said that the decrease of diphtheria for 1960 has been 60% in comparison to 1959 but what the morbidity of it was in either year they do not tell. For the same years the corresponding figure for polio is 44%. It is claimed that the incidence also of Brucellosis, pertussis, venereal diseases, trachoma and fifteen other infectious diseases has considerably subsided. The subsidence of tuberculosis amounts to 3½ times that of 1959.

General mortality in 1960 was 7.2%. The first place in it is occupied by the cardio-vascular diseases. This is a direct denunciation of the theory of dialectics and Nervism since in the capitalistic American world the first place is also held by the same diseases.

The birth rate in the USSR is unknown to us, though sources exist from which we could find it. The birth rate has the top Party and Medical leaders openly worried, because of the decline. The reason is not only the generations which perished in World War II, nor is it only the low standard of living. We have the clear impression that the Party oppression, the indoctrination practiced and, most of all, the discrepancy between what is preached and what the realities are with the thorny privileges of the Party members, contribute to the prevailing small size of the Soviet family. The same is true regarding each of the satellites where people oppose the Party in every way they can without getting into obvious trouble.

At the same time the family size in the U.S.A. is much greater than in any other of the civilized nations. Here also it is not the economic factor that is the primary cause. The background is the respected dignity of man, the true democracy in the nation and the higher sense of sacrifice, of service. The high birth rate is of vital importance because in the future more and more the number of the masses will be a determining factor in the entire national and international relationship and life. Unfortunately in the U.S. legislation is urgently needed to ensure healthy generations. This will contribute more to the growth of the nation, growth which is faster than that of the USSR.

The death rate of infants in the USSR is 36 per 1000 live births. This is a figure which is much higher than in the U.S. where it is at the level of 25. Here is how the problem is put by the president of the American Academy of Pediatrics:

"We are also concerned with the national picture of infant mortality, which has leveled off in recent years after a rapid decline in the rate during the 1940's. A recent able analysis shows that the situation is largely due to our inability to affect any reduction in neonatal deaths. The percentage of deaths under one month of age has also shown a tendency to increase in some states and in certain groups of the population." (Dr. G. M. Wheatley, Presidential Address; *The Academy* 1960-1961, *Pediatrics*, Jan. 1, 1962).

The same causes of infant mortality are pointed out in the USSR, but there the fight against it resembles a crusade which is requiring the efforts of every patriot in every part of the country. Following is the spirit and nuance of Dr. Wheatley, president of the American Academy of Pediatrics, in which he formulates the obligations:

". . . it seems timely to remind ourselves that the hallmark of our specialty since its inception has been involvement in community service . . . Everyone can exercise this kind of leadership. If we do, the future growth of the Academy is secure." (Ibid.)

PART V

SUMMARIES AND CONCLUSIONS

SUMMARIES AND CONCLUSIONS

VIRTUES OF SOVIET MEDICINE

1. In one sense, Soviet medicine is, above all, a practical science. It is fully dedicated to the welfare of the individual and of society. Formally, it is free to the individual in health, disaster or need. The government is spending tremendous sums of money mostly for the advancement of the medical sections of the health organization. Hospitals are overstaffed with medical personnel. The administrative section is much smaller and unconditionally subordinated to the medical hierarchy. It is not suffocated by additional services independent of the doctor on the spot. Attempts are being made to alleviate the great expenditures by means of a simpler method of carrying out health services. Economy is an utmost primacy. Increasing efforts are made for the invention of, or supply from abroad, of modern drugs and equipment. Physiotherapy of all kinds is underlined by the same considerations, and is superdeveloped and practiced more than in any other country.

2. Soviet medicine is attempting, and has succeeded, in reaching the entire life of the individuals and the society, including part of their education. It has not left without attention any medical aspect of human nature. This is especially true of children. In this respect, much is being contributed by the optimistic and high humanitarian teaching of Pavlov.

Numerous scientists, doctors and experimenters work along the lines paved by Pavlov and are attempting to reveal the physiological, and, therefore, pedagogical and psychological mechanisms in the formation of the individual. Of course this is being done to benefit the Party in its domination, but people and the vast number of intellectuals including teachers will, for the most part, adjust all, more or less, according to their tastes. For this reason, in the long run especially, it will have a most beneficial effect on youth and society. For while the Russians have their unopposed, almighty God, Pavlov that is positive science, U.S. medicine has no one in particular, and its psychiatry recognizes Freud who is incompatible with Christ and science. They have almost maniacal tendencies in building, constructing, reforming, educating and preventing diseases. *The prophylactic trend is the most conspicuous and powerful trend of Soviet medicine.*

3.   An immense number of people are involved in research and carrying out the medical services. The very great number of doctors is fast increasing. Now there are about 400,000   In the U.S. there are less than 270,000. In 1960, the USSR graduated 26,000 young specialists *(Vestnik Akademii Meditsinskih Nauk of USSR,* #9, 1961).

According to John Gunther nearly 1% of the population of the USSR is involved in one way or another in service in the fields of health *(Inside Russia Today,* London, 1958).

4.   Another fundamental virtue of Russian medicine dominated by Pavlov's teaching is the philosophy of responsibility of the individual. This philosophy greatly benefits society and also the individual, directly and indirectly. The opinion of Professor Milton

Senn (Yale University, a visitor to the USSR) that "The Russians see little need for help from psychologists, psychiatrists or other social scientists in the rearing of children and in the helping of those who are having difficulties in learning, obeying, following orders or in other ways of performing," points out only a natural sequel of the above Russian philosophy. By revealing the conflicts of personality under Communism, those good specialists would not at all cause the Party to drop Communism. They would only spoil the individual by weakening his will and increasing the overall pathology. So the adherence to Pavlov's teaching and to the philosophy of responsibility is observed not only because of fear on anyone's part but also because, as Gaylord says, it was rooted by nature. Conversely, the philosophy of irresponsibility on the grounds of Freudism, Lobrozianism is deteriorating society as well as the individual. The philosophy of the irresponsibility of the individual, hidden behind Freudism and other "bio-social" concepts, is from a true biological and social point of view, a real venom to the sound forces promoting life, that is, survival, progress, freedom and happiness. How responsibility is preached in the Soviet Union by the medical people is evidenced in some degree only from the following citations from the speech of the Soviet minister of Public Health.

"In several fields we are still lagging behind the most advanced capitalistic countries . . . Activity of the Academy of Medical Sciences of USSR will be concentrated basically to the development of mathematical, humanitarian and natural sciences . . . The cost of hospitalizing a patient in our Research institutes amounts to 1½ that in other first class hospitals. Is there any sense in using the money in such irrational manner? To many of those present here it is known that in the U.S. the national heart institute or the cancer institute largely use various hospitals for carrying on those clinical investigations. . . . The whole job on tuberculosis for instance and other clinical problems is carried on in the hospitals where doctors are attracted for that purpose and are practicing in these same hospitals. We ought to take this into consideration.

"Every year international scientific communications increase, the number of the countries unselfishly helped by the Soviet Union grows . . . The coefficient of usefulness of our scientific workers when they are on missions abroad is reduced because of their ignorance of foreign languages . . . We must pay very serious attention to the language preparedness of our youth at the institutions of the Academy. We cannot rest with this, that persons who have embraced science are not in command of even one foreign language.

". . . with the use of foreign literature on a large scale at times confusion arises, and frequently works of hostile ideology and doubtful in scientific sense penetrate our country. . . . Coexistence not only does not reject but presumes the continuation of the ideological struggle . . . (C. V. Kurashov, Minister of Public Health, *Herald of Academy of Medical Science* AMS of USSR #9, 1961).

5. Another paramount virtue of Soviet medicine is the very great degree of dedication. It has such a dedi-

cation because it has an ideal. It is in constant aggression for this ideal which is the nationalistic-chauvinistic-ideological goal of the very Communist Party. The USSR is an empire without parallel in history. There are more than 160 languages spoken, most of them having nothing in common. Over one third of the population is of non-Slavic origin, and territories have been "united" and subordinated through unprecedented bloodshed. The history of the Moscow kingship and its rise to the present state is something which has never occurred elsewhere on the globe. It caused more suffering and death to people of all races than the Communist counterpart, — the Nazi, — succeeded in inflicting upon the Jewish nationality. Nevertheless the Communists ultimately achieved a greater success. This endows the Russians with special pride and privileges. At the same time the horrid Communist regime and the Iron Curtain for decades has been keeping them isolated, blamed and inferior. This makes them all feel injured and they are eager and mad to prove to the entire world and especially to the Americans what they really are and what their classical Gogol meant in describing one of his romantic characters of the 16th Century.

This hero was caught by the Poles because he was unwilling to let them get his pipe that fell while being pursued. He stopped, got down off the horse and searched for the pipe in the grass. So the Poles caught him and "fastened him with iron chains to the trunk of the tree and drove nails into his hands . . . beneath they piled fagots . . . the flames rose, gripping his feet and running up the tree." But what force on earth can be found to overpower his power! He, after instructing by loud cries his endangered and pursued comrades, says his last words to the Poles. "Wait. The day will come when you shall learn what the Orthodox Russian is! Already people far and near forebode it: There shall arise a ruler from the Russian soil, and there shall be no power on earth that shall not yield to him." Naturally by "on earth" he meant the world known to his epoch. But the important thing here is his determination and his faith and spirit.

Of course, such a powerful drive could not evolve otherwise. Of a similar spirit is the intensive and ceaseless Communist propaganda on patriotism. To be successful it transforms itself in the fashion fitting history and evolution itself. This fashion proved to be Communism. Russian Communists now are carrying on the drive to conquer the world. In this process Soviet medicine is an active, deliberate and formidable participant. From the point of view of the Russian interests and pride, Soviet medicine is a power and organization of great virtue.

THE HANDICAPS OF SOVIET MEDICINE

From what was already said regarding Soviet medicine, it will suffice to briefly enumerate its fundamental handicaps.

1. The great majority of its cadres are poorly selected and trained, exhausted by para-medical indoctrination and formalistic obligations. They are devoid of creative spirit and imagination because of poverty, injustices of the Party and lack of freedom. That is why Soviet medicine will continue, for a long time to come, trailing scientifically far behind the medicine of the U.S. That it is correct is sufficiently elicited by the following observations:

"To the Americans," writes British Dr. Horman, "who originate and have the first trial of many more things than we do, they (the Russians) would seem even more behind time.

"What struck me about medical Russia was the Englishness of it all," in fact, its Americanness, as far as it is simulating mainly American medical science, in theory and practice.

"No doubt their patients are under-investigated by American standards," continues Dr. Horman, "and under-treated.

"In the clinical field, I hardly found a single new idea, — good, bad, provocative, ingenius, fantastic or even silly, but," says Dr. Horman,

"They were proud of what they were doing and were anxious to show it. The exception to this sameness is psychiatric medicine. Freud's views are anathema, being 'idealistic.' I conclude that Russian internal medicine is a faithful copy of our own, and I see no point in thinking of Russia as a place of medical pilgrimage."

Thus ends the extraordinarily true evaluations of this British doctor who is nearer to Russia than the Americans who are shocked by the "unusual achievements" of Soviet medicine.

2. The role of the Party has been positive in the practical field of carrying out medical services to the needs of society. In the scientific field, the detrimental overall role of the Party has prevailed. This has occurred because of the unlimited interference of the Party in the scientific thinking and practice. For medicine is something more than a pure, complex science. It is as much a creative and inspiring art which

can flourish best in the climate of freedom, security and happiness as conceived and felt by the doctors, not by the Party.

3. Soviet medicine, as represented by its post-revolution cadres and complex elements is a product and a part of the Party itself with its interference through privileges, injustices, and terror, and cannot exist in its present form without the support of the Communist regime. It, therefore, is an artificial creation devoid of self-confidence, honesty, creative imagination and invention. Its moving force, the doctor, is overloaded with paper work, humiliation and tremendous and exhausting trivial daily labor and obligations imposed by the Party.

4. Soviet medicine is the most wasteful and expensive in the world. Boasts on the part of the Communist propagandists that it is free of any charge for the vast masses of the people is not true. This is so because, first, drugs are a monopoly of the government and are sold at prices that bring about great profits. Secondly, because the standard of living determined by the same Communist Government is three to five times lower than in many Western countries and especially in the U.S. Equally groundless is the pretense that Soviet medicine is based on the principle of the family doctor. In fact, they are only attempting this.

5. Soviet medicine is paying great homage to specialization. All their doctors tend to specialize. This makes the medical practice too complicated, bureaucratic and troublesome for the people. Besides, it automatically abolishes to a great extent the principle of the family doctor the Communists aim at keeping.

6. In comparison with the vast sums of money spent and the research done, it is sterile and up to the

present it has not achieved one invention or epochal discovery. In this respect Russian pre-Revolution medicine is far superior to the post-Revolution Soviet medicine. In fact, Soviet medicine has been an impudent boaster and at the same time a shameless and ungrateful consumer of the achievements of Western, and mainly American, medicine. Characteristic of it also is its philosophical speculations and perversiveness.

7. Soviet medicine does not possess the qualities of an original school, specific of USSR, even though adhering strictly to Pavlov's teaching and negating Freud.

8. A trait of Soviet medicine which has been paid no attention but potentially is of ominous significance is the hyperaggressiveness. It is second only to that of the Communist Party. This is true to an extent of wildness and its interpretation would be most just if we confine it to what is known as vulgar biologism. It has been and is flourishing under the pressure and rivalry of the Party, no matter how paradoxical this may seem. As a response to the insecurity and the threat of the Party which is the factor distributing the loaf of bread, Soviet medics are developing tremendous aggressive drives, grabbing greater and greater perimeter of their society. The most recent incursion is upon children. The latter are encompassed in a galloping speed by the care of psychiatrists, no matter if they are of Pavlovian zest. This practically is only another version of what is going on in the West and especially in the U.S. Soon the professional "competence" and "concern" will start producing psychotics and fostering them to the detriment of the entire society. Yes, human nature is everywhere the same, regardless of the "colors" . . .

The Weak Points Of American Medicine

These weak points are four.

1. *Freudism* on which we have sufficiently elaborated.

2. *The high cost* to the people. It is true that real, successful medicine such as creates epochs in history, is inconsistent with poverty, with a situation in which the doctor is a type of poor society servant or hard worker as he is in the USSR; it needs the air of freedom, security, self-confidence and that material basis which gives wings for every progress and high horizon.

Alas, the costliness of U.S. medicine is not compatible with the cry of our epoch, or even with the very interests of the medical profession. It is therefore high time that something be done on the part of all involved in the practice of medicine. The recently discussed medical aid for the aged is only one of the phenomena characteristic of our time. We do not mean socialization at all. For socialized medicine, as we pointed out elsewhere, is not only not cheap but, in fact, very costly and of low scientific and moral standard. But we are of the sincere opinion that our system of free enterprise is facing such ideological perils that if we do not undertake convincing steps to show its superiority over the ideologies of demagogy and slavery, we all will inevitably lose everything. We must work more and produce more thus we will have more beds and better care for all.

3. *The Mental Hospitals.* They are the black and tragic portions in the fascinating kaleidoscope of U.S. medicine. It is not only because they have more or less Freudian handling of the patients or because of their ominous number, — 25 for instance, in Ohio alone,

whose population is nine million, thus dooming to neglect the remaining first class problems of society. They have become an independent empire with departments resembling kingships. While every other institution including the governorship is subjected to tight control and regeneration after a short span of electorial life, the leadership of the mental hospitals is something more stable and independent than the top executive of the state. The only thing which the leadership of the mental hospital know best is not more work, sacrifice and economy, but to always cry for more credits, to always lament about being neglected. The administrative sector on its part has shown incontrolability in its drive to expand and expend. Thus the vital medical factor is suffocating because of inadequate appropriations. At the same time it has abdicated from its responsibility for being the main factor, in favor of the maintenance and administrative sectors, to the encouragement of bureaucratism and waste.

The mental hospital leadership is, it seems, unconcerned about the urgent need of a reappraisal, reorganization and rationalization of mental hospital realities. Everybody associated with those hospitals sees the backwardness and the waste. It is time for every American to rise and crusade against this unfortunate side of our free society.

The politicians feel the backwardness, they are eager to introduce reforms, but do not possess the competence to strike the blow regardless of the resistance. The specialists, lacking the ideal, the responsibility, and driven by the forces of the vulgar and primitive biologism, have one goal only, to not only retain their present empire of bureaucracy but to expand it, thus more and more placing society in a helpless situation of financial and political crisis.

4. *The lack of ideal* is the paramount inferiority of U.S. medicine. With this lack of ideal actually Freudism, costliness and retardation of mental hospitals are linked. We do not mean that U.S. medicine should search for a new ideal. We have it and it is ever new, — the Ideal of Christianity. Not without justification is medical aid identified with the Good Samaritan from the Holy Gospel. What we need is to realize the necessity for a new presentation of the great Christian ideal which cannot be better expressed by any other human discipline than by medicine. Medicine is the synthesis of almost all of the remaining sciences including the philosophy of morality. In other words, medicine can justly be called a practical Christianity. Well, such a vocation cannot be contradictory to itself, to ignore the social and political realities and allow our ideal to be beaten every day by Communism. For we may consider this ideal of Communism as a caricature, one which never can be fulfilled, one which a few only believe can be attained, one which is incompatible with human freedom and man's evolutionally established rights and feelings. But we are in the 20th century, now in the space age. The masses became bold and pretentious, smart, and are now transferring the warfare from between themselves to oppose any conservatism, injustice and egoism. This is not an accidental or ephemeral phenomenon; it is a profound evolutionary, revolutionary change. Now there are pros and cons, East and West; they are divided and sooner or later the final fateful battle will take place between them. Here the number of the masses will play a decisive role. Whoever remains alone or with

few friends will be defeated. If we wish, therefore, to be the victorious counterpart, we must win the masses, the peoples throughout the globe. But we can do that, not mainly by money or by preaching abroad one philosophy while at home we follow another. We must have ideals, an ideology appealing enough to defeat Communism. Unfortunately up to the present we have not shown that we realize this vital fact.

The consequences of this are relevant to us all, — our country, our families, ourselves. We, American medics, therefore, cannot afford to stay inactive at a time when the Communist doctors-academicians are waging an all out ideological offensive against the very substance and existence of our world.

THE GREAT VIRTUES OF U.S. MEDICINE

We have to continue the appraisal of American Medicine by resorting to an excursion into some information dating three decades ago.

Dr. Vassil Zonchev was the most outstanding pupil of Professor Vassil Mollov, known in his native country as the Bulgarian "Friedrich Muller." Zonchev now is professor at the State University of Sofia, the capital of Bulgaria. In the mid-thirties he visited the U.S. and remained for nearly one year. He knew English very well, and similarly French, German and Russian. Before coming to the U.S., he had attended many international congresses and on several occasions visited Germany, Austria, France and Italy. His favorite medical periodicals in English were the *JAMA* and the *Archives of Internal Medicine*. His most esteemed English book on internal diseases was Osler-Christian's work and his desk reference book on pathological and normal physiology was Best and Taylor's *Physiological Basis of Medical Practice.*

On his return to Bulgaria in 1938, he gave an in- • formative lecture before the Sofia Society of Internists. His reports of American medicine of that time were, generally, very unfavorable. As an exception he mentioned Johns Hopkins Hospital, the Mayo Clinics and Chicago. To us who were friends of America it was a bitter disappointment. During the war the story of Penicillin stirred us up as previously we had been moved by the victory over malaria in the Pacific Islands which had affected such a large percentage of American combatant troops.

Immediately following World War II, we were continuously impressed by the achievements in American medicine and very frequently commented and shared whatever information any of us had. Here I recollect what one of our friends, a colleague trained in Germany and Austria, an eminent cardiologist in Sofia, Dr. Pastuhov, said regarding U.S. medicine:

> "In the twenties, Americans who came as visitors or to specialize in Vienna were not paid any serious attention by the professors but were left to the assistants. Later on," Dr. Pastuhov continued, "the Austrian professors became more impressed by the preparedness of the Americans and looked upon them as their favorites. Still later," he concluded, "the Americans were lecturing and the Austrian clinicians-professors were listening to them with respect and praise." This all occurred in less than twenty years!

A few months ago, drawn by the image of the U.S.A., there came to this country another physician, a specialist, Dr. X, educated in Germany and France. He knows German, French and Russian very well, has participated in international congresses and is the author of a number of scientific papers and other works. Here is his reply to our appeal to him to share his impressions of American medicine as compared with the Soviet medicine which he has followed for over two decades:

"1.   The practicality of American medicine in the sense that treatment is carried on with unusual preciseness and clarity, thanks to the full use of all modern investigations, tests and clinical observations. Treatment is undertaken in the shortest possible time following the patient's hospitalization, in the greatest safety and comfort for him. Clinical medicine has accepted the laboratory and relies upon it; Americans are the only ones making full and gratifying use of this resource.

"2.   The great number of synthetic and efficient preparations amazes every European doctor. The effectiveness and the clinical life of a part of them will surely be well known later, but the fact of the availability of all of them cannot but evoke the admiration of every doctor.

"3.   The question arises as to why American medicine is far ahead of the Russian. It is because under Communism the individual and his human personality are unimportant creations; they are only a part of the government machinery and an instrument of the Party. The physician has no other choice but to comply with the Party and its ideological line and be an impersonal part of the same government machinery.

"4.   The entire medical education in the USSR is organized and set in such a way that more than one third of the subjects are of a mere military and political nature. The Party wants the physician to be a ready soldier for the war through which Communism plans to impose its rule over the world. This is all carried on to the detriment of the medical education.

"5.   Free health service is one of the ways the poor Soviet citizens are kept in abeyance. Simultaneously this free health service is a propaganda weapon. Yet much of the expense for the health service is covered by the profits the Government obtains from the monopoly on the production and sale of drugs; it is the people who pay all . . .

"6.   A characteristic of Russian doctors is that they speculate too much. They persistently attempt to adjust everything to their theories of Marxism and Nervism and do not follow the language of the facts. The Party tyrannizes the doctors, who, in return, to survive, deceive the Party, the people and the world. In this the Russian medical profession presents a sharp contrast to the American doctors whose honesty, regard for truth and whose precise analysis of the facts without any prejudice are so typical of American medicine and lie at the root of its almost unbelievable progress.

"7.   Soviet medicine has been unable to give mankind even one great invention, though it had full access to Western and American achievements and ideas. If they have any such invention it is a secret, which by itself is immoral. Sterility, philo-

sophy and impudent boasts are the most characteristic of Soviet medics, because, being sterile
and yet obligated to the Party for privileges while
at the same time they feared the tyranny of the
Party, Soviet doctors and academicians had to resort to this methodology of talkativeness, boasts
and plagiarism. Another reason is that they explain all of man's pathology on the basis of Nervism which is an absurdity.

"8. Ignoring the facts and wandering into un-
certainties, Soviet clinicians and scientists have
no other choice but to speak of generalities, obscure judgments and explanations, thus often resembling the Scholastics of the middle centuries.

"9. It should be pointed out that generally,
articles appearing in Soviet journals as original,
frequently are but repetition of what was published or had happened in the West, and especially
in the U.S. Problems and ideas which are discussed and published in the U.S. one can trace in
Soviet literature months later. This is a truth recognized by every one who is cognizant of Soviet
medical science. While doing this, Soviet authors
in most cases mention nothing with respect to the
American sources and authors who originated the
ideas or discoveries."

Another, Dr. Y, assistant professor at the University
of Warsaw, who left Poland about three years ago and
is now a resident of the U.S., shared with us this opinion with respect to Soviet and American medicine.

"1. Soviet medicine has shown greatest progress in the field of public health and epidemiology,
the field which has been conquered a long time

ago by the American doctor, society and free social order.

"2.   In the realm of real medical science and
research, Soviet medicine is retarded. The reason
for this is the oppression by the Party, and the
poverty of the Soviet doctor. Only the academicians and those with various titles and 'merits'
have pay sufficient to have a satisfactory living.
Because of the unattractive status of the Soviet
doctor, brilliant people rarely embrace the medical profession and thus Soviet medical cadres
are generally lacking gifted people.

"3.   Typical of Soviet medicine is the over-em-
phasized Pavlovism (Nervism).

"4.   Soviet medicine is virtually copying the
ideas and thematics of Western and American medicine. The only original and useful thing I
learned from Soviet medicine was the delivery
pain prophylaxy which consists of suggestion, that
is of discourse with the pregnant woman and convincing her that she will not experience pain while
giving birth to a child. This method, based again
on Nervism, works to some extent in some instances only, and is impractical on a large scale at
a maternity hospital.

"5.   American medicine as judged by me: In
Warsaw I was one of the first; here I am one of
the last.

"6.   To the question: What new drugs have
the Soviet Union academicians and research scientists discovered for the benefit of suffering mankind? The answer is: Absolutely none."

AMERICAN MEDICAL ACHIEVEMENTS SUMMARIZED

That these doctors are just in their appraisals you can estimate and judge for yourself when you know that the progress of modern medicine is mostly by American merit. For example:

Much new clinical nomenclature, such as Fibro-elastosis, Toxoplasmosis, Fibrocystic disease, Hyaline Membrane disease, Coxsackie infections, many syndromes, etc., etc.

The new methodology of heart pathology diagnostics and heart surgery.

The epochal invention of the antibiotics of varying spectrum and of varying duration of activity.

The classification of the collagen diseases and the prevention of acute rheumatic fever.

The dramatic victory of the treatment and the prevention of the two most dangerous venereal diseases.

The attempt at control of malignancies by a series of new drugs.

The new methods of early diagnosis of malignancies in the genycological area.

The finding of the Rh factor with all subsequent widening of the field of blood pathology and physiology.

The life saving anticoagulant therapy whose substance was discovered by an American medical student.

The vitally important knowledge of the electrolyte correlations and their applications in man's pathology.

Brain tumor surgery and the surgery of brain blood vessels.

The new cardio-vascular drugs, the anti-athero-matosis drugs, the new anti-hypertensive drugs and the diuretics of non-mercurial nature.

The discovery of the Adrenocorticotropic hormone and of the corticosteroids with their wide significance in modern therapeutics.

The anti-convulsive drugs, the tranquilizers and anti-depressants, all considered by some as "miraculous."

The new understanding of diabetes and the new methods of investigation and controlling it.

The new achievements in the field of endocrinology, liver pathology and congenital diseases.

The polio vaccines of Dr. Salk and Dr. Sabin.

The newest trend of mass vaccination against tuberculosis even though it is disappearing in the U.S. We hope that when this report is in the hands of the reader we will have ready a measles vaccine, and effective cold vaccine.

The new tests and laboratory methods that tremendously increase the efficiency of the clinics.

The list could be greatly increased but it will suffice if the reader will think only of the recent number of Nobel prize-winning American scientists in the medico-biological field, and that there is not one Russian.

In less than four decades the U.S. medicine acquired the physiognomy of highest ranking medical school with much specific science, methodology and achievements.

Naturally a complex of factors underlies the unusually fast progress and achievements of United States medical science. No other nation or scientific field of such magnitude has ever in history demonstrated such a feat. It is worthy of pointing out some of the propelling forces of its progress.

1.   In the first place there is the climate of the great freedom which gives wings to every progress and creativity. This great freedom comprises the value of man, the scientist, — his security and self-confidence, his inspiration and intellectual-spiritual balance and his material welfare.

2.   The building up of the cadre body by means of true natural selection. The great prosperity does not favor mediocrities and the latter are not being pushed ahead by a Party through fidelity to the ideology. Thus, in the U.S. generally only intellectual-moral superiors have been entering the scientific field of medicine and they manifest their capacities and morality in science in a manner recognized by all throughout the globe.

3.   The private contributions on the part of great patriots, the industrialists and people of every walk of life who, of their own free will, contribute immensely to the progress of pure medical science, unpoisoned by any interference.

Similar revelations of this erection of U.S. medicine are brought out by the thoughts of Lord Taylor, M.D., in his article, *Dynamics of American Medicine, (Lancet,* February 21, 1959, p. 705).

"We may think that the ordinary people of Britain get better deals from our National health service than the ordinary people get in America. We may think we suffer less from social neuroses, etc., but in the advancement of medical practice and research we have definitely fallen behind them."

These comments Lord Taylor makes in conjunction

with the autobiography of *Dr. Leonard G. Rowntree.*
The eminent British doctor (Lord Taylor) goes on
thus:

"So he (Rowntree) has made his autobiography a
biographical history of the 20th century medicine.
Such a book could hardly have been written by a
retired English consultant, for it has a splendid lack
of reticence. This clinical truthfulness is perhaps the
first secret of American medical success. Everyone
has got to stand up to criticism. With the lack of
reticence goes a freedom from cynicism, malice and
uncharitableness. There are three places where modern American medicine has been forged . . . The
Johns Hopkins Hospital, The Mayo Clinic and the
Rockefeller Institute. Now, of course, their influence
has spread far and wide."

"Yes," once Ernest Renan said:

"No great moral thought could proceed from races
oppressed by secular despotism, and accustomed to
institutions which precluded the exercise of individual
liberty." And medicine is a moral science also.

Another striking trait of superiority and virtue of
American medicine is its methodology. In learning
and in teaching, in using sources and in writing theory
and in practice, in carrying on differential diagnosis
and in search of diagnosis, the American doctor and
student of medicine are always exemplary. They are
not poisoned by Marxian doctrinairism, that is, phi-
losophies, boastful slogans, speculations and obscurities often covering ignorance, helplessness and dishonesty. American medicine works with concrete
elements and pursues concrete goals, with no waste
of time, piously obedient to the hard facts. It talks
little and it does great.

American doctors have displayed two other virtues unmatched by adherents of Aesculapius in any other country of the world. One unrecognized and unnoticed virtue of American doctors is their altruistic treatment of their foreign colleagues. The latter, as DP's, — refugees, escapees from Communism or choosers of America for other reasons, are received with kindness and help as brothers. After one or two years of some fruitful hardships they acquire the right to make their living at a level undreamed of in any other nation in the world.

The other American virtue is the doctors' unusual faithfulness to the basic national institutions and ideas. No American doctor ever conspired against the liberties and the order of his country. His counterparts all over the world have been involved in anti-Government activities in percentage only equalled by the lawyers, agronomists and teachers. Prior to the enslavement of the "Satellites," the doctors there were the leading anti-Government intelligentsia portion of Communists. Of course, following the Communist take-over there under the protection of the Soviet tank divisions and NVD, their "idealism" was confined to their becoming bosses of the masses, to taking high post without having the proper qualifications and to grabbing privileges without justification.

In summing up, it is not only the riches; the unbelievable private contributions and esteem of medicine; the nobleness; the humility and sense of fidelity to the heritage and the welfare of the nation; the honesty and devotion to duty; the hard work which Osler considered "the master-word in medicine." It is a product of all these virtues. What makes it all the more remarkable and worthy of every admiration is that all this was mostly attained for such a short time. Russian medicine in forty-five years and despite the incomparably great government support in funds and man power and the unlimited and timely access to American medicine and medical ideas, did not achieve any scientific distinction. And if Soviet medicine did not use the contributions and progress of Western, and especially American, medicine, at what point would it be now? American medicine never resorted to Soviet medical knowledge! It did use Russian medical science prior to the October Revolution, for Russian pre-Revolution medicine was outstanding and its standard was never reached by Communist medicine.

Modest, profoundly democratic, honest, working unpretentiously in search for means against disease, unhappiness and death the American doctor has, together with his great, noble nation, to be proud of the achievements and contributions to the treasury of American medical science to which humanity owes so much for its welfare and happiness. Such is the American doctor because he has behind him the great Christian spirit of his generous nation: they have never done anything wrong to any people, they rather have tried to serve all mankind.

What a sharp contrast the American doctor is, compared to the Soviet doctor-scientist-academician! Just imagine what occurred in the USSR during and following the revolution! It all is partially described by Sholohov, Veressaev, the literature of the escapees from behind the Iron Curtain and by Mr. Khrushchev himself. There is no comparable tragedy in history. The crimes of Caligula or Robespierre are a petite episode in comparison with the dreadful crimes of Stalin.

Again he was the object of glorification and deification by whom? By the Communist Party and by the Soviet doctor-scientist-academicians! How did it all occur? Thanks to the Party itself, to the Party historical background reaching back to Ivan the Terrible, the Oprichina and the anti-Semitism.

The Soviet medics, instead of showing repentance and feeling shame and disgrace, as we have documentarily pointed out in this work, are waging a permanent ideological warfare against freedom, with the intention of destroying our world and replacing it with theirs!

According to them, — the Soviet coryphaei of medicine, academicians and Communist doctors, — we are doomed and they are just helping history and evolution complete the liquidation. All Soviet scientists mean, in their speeches of friendship or hatred, in their smiles of coexistence or of superiority, in their wild ideological and "scientific" assaults against the free world, in all they do at home or abroad, officially or not, they aim at speeding up our burial. These truths must be as clear to the American doctors as 2 plus 2 equals 4. American doctors, and first of all their leadership in the AMA, must realize these realities and their implications.

The Power of New Ideas

Despite the indescribable crimes and anti-human nature of Communism, it appeals very highly because of its novelty in the centuries-old miserable grayness of the masses, because of their distance from its realities, but mostly because of its promises. New, promising ideas always have been more powerful than money, physical or military might. Christ offered the

reward and promise of the Kingdom of God alone and
He conquered the world. Of course, barbarians have
also "conquered" the world through their mightier
drives (primitive ideas), because of a lack of ideals
on the part of the defeated, or at least their failure to
fight for their ideals. Americans have far more original
higher ideas than the Russians. The tragedy is that
they, the Americans, do not find it vital to persist and
fight for these ideas, or they do that insufficiently.

FINDING AND FIGHTING FOR OUR IDEALS

What is our ideal, and where shall we look for it?
There are two places to seek for it. The one is Christ's
teaching in its unsurpassable and eternal grandeur of
symbolization of higher happiness. The other is the domain of natural sciences, according to which (Pavlov,
for instance) freedom is an indispensable premise of
happiness. According to the same natural sciences
(Darwin) only he who is stronger than his enemies
can secure freedom for himself. Happiness through
freedom in the broadest sense of the term, therefore,
must be our ideal. In the pursuit of this ideal who is
more obligated and able to make a greater scientific
investment and contribute a larger share than medicine
and doctors? Almost none.

Here we come across Communism as an adverse
ideal of ours. For this its adherents of all walks of
life are in permanent mobilization of all their intellectual and physical power aimed at our total destruction. Soviet doctors also fervidly seek the attainment
of the same ideal.

It is more than clear that to counteract this drive of
Communism we must work for our ideal with greater

dedication, fighting spirit, and faithfulness than the Communists work for their ideal. To carry on this fateful task we have all the material and intellectual power, the history, the natural sciences and Christ. But this we have been possessing already and yet we are the losers. Why? The answer is easy to give: because our enemy persisted in remaining a real enemy of ours and faithful to his ideals while we did not. This weakens us, downgrades and alienates us from our old allies and friends and prevents us from gaining new ones.

The inference is simple. We either have to resume combating and standing for our ideal or we will become alone and perish altogether in a most dishonorable manner. This must be well remembered by the politicians who are betraying freedom, that is our vital ideal; by those of the Holy Fathers who are extending their hand to the Devil (Communism) and by these Christians who believe that God will grant them happiness and freedom, not through the fulfillment of His natural laws but through some sort of miracle. Doctors, being naturalists, must not forget that down to the minutest molecular level, *life is change*. The same is true of ideas. It is through them that "the first become last and the last, first." Doctors must help our statesmen who are failing because of their super-kindness toward the enemy. It is only through political science that the moral and scientific progress can be fully applied to life. It is absurd for doctors to think that they and their nation can indefinitely be secure in their present freedom, prosperity and scientific progress while ignoring the new ideas of higher humanitarianism.

American doctors dare not one day longer ignore

such devastating threats to the physical, mental and moral health of the nation as racial discrimination, criminal, decadent and ugly literature and art, rising delinquency, lagging education with its loss of talent, unemployment with its demoralizing effects and subversive role of "welfare" services and on the world front, ignorance, misery and slavery under Communism. This is all a horrible injustice with which we must *never* be reconciled. For Thomas Jefferson said, "I tremble for my country when I reflect that God is just."

BIBLIOGRAPHY

(Only a part of Russian sources in translation are given.)

1. *Herald of the Academy of Medical Sciences of USSR*, No. 5, 1956, No. 1-12, 1960, 1961 and Jan., Feb., March, and April, 1962.

2. *Journal of the Higher Nervous Activity*, No. 6, Vol. 6, 1956.

3. *Journal of Neuropathology and Psychiatry for the Name of S.S. Korssakov*, No. 9-12 1959, No. 1-12, 1960, 1961, and Jan., Feb., March, April, and May, 1962.

4. *Klinical Medicine*, No. 1-12, 1960, 1961, and Jan., Feb., March, April, and May, 1962.

5. *Pediatria*, No. 1-12, 1957, 1958, 1959, 1960, 1961 and Jan., Feb., March and April, 1962.

6. *Problems in Protection of Motherhood and Childhood*, No. 1-12, 1957, 1958, 1959, 1960, 1961 and Jan., Feb., March, April, and May, 1962.

7. *Problems of Tuberculosis*, No. 1-12, 1957, 1958, 1959, 1960, 1961, and Jan., Feb., March, April, and May, 1962.

8. Ado, A.D., *The Immunological Processes as a Total Reaction of the Organism, Etc. Contemporary Medicine* No. 3, 1952, Sofia.

9. Ablaev, E.M., *Transfusions to Tuberculous Patients, Problems of Tuberculosis* No. 1, 1955.

10. Asseev, D.D., *Principles and Methods of Treatment Tuberculous Patients, Soviet Medicine* No. 8, 1955.

11. Baranov, V.G., *Contemporary Problems of Epidemiology in the Light of the Teaching of I.P. Pavlov, Therapeutic Archives* No. 1, 1951.

12. Bilibin, A.F., *Ways of the Reconstruction of the Teaching of Infectious Diseases upon the Basic Conditions of the Pavlovian Trend in Medicine, Contemporary Medicine* No. 3, 1951, Sofia.

13. Birukov, D.A., *I. P. Pavlov, Moscow, Academy of Medical Science of the USSR*, 1949.

14. Bookin, V.N., *Vitamins, Moscow-Leningrad*, 1940.

15. Chernigovsky, V.N., *The Prophylactic Trend of Medicine, Etc., Problems of Tuberculosis*, No. 1, 1956.

16. Dobrohvalov, V.P., *Philosophical and Natural Sciences Premises of the Teaching of I.P. Michurin, Soviet Science*, Moscow, 1954.

17. Dombrovaska, U.F., *Pneumonias of Early Childhood*, Third Ed., 1955.

309

18. Education: *The Teaching of I. P. Pavlov in the Theoretical and Practical Medicine,* Second Volume, 1953, Moscow.

19. Gogol, N.V., *Taras Bulba,* Foreign Languages Publishing House, Moscow. Gogol, N.V., *Dead Souls,* Foreign Languages Publishing House, Moscow.

20. Greenchar, N.N., *Tuberculosis of the Lungs,* Moscow, 1947.

21. Ivanov, A.G., Smolensky, *Essays on the Patho-Physiology of the Higher Nervous Activity,* Moscow, Foreign Languages Publishing House, 1954.

22. Langovoy, N., Vlassov V., and Blinder D., *A Textbook of Diseases of Children* MEDGIS, Moscow, 1945.

23. Masslov, M.S., *Diseases of Children,* Second Ed., Leningrad, MEDGIS, 1946.

24. Model, L.M., *The Contemporary Condition of the Immunological Problems in Tuberculosis — Problems of Tuberculosis,* No. 4, 1950.

25. Olevsky, M.I., *Effect of Varying Contents of Protein in Nutrition Upon the Development and Function of the Growing Child Organism,* Works VI. *All-Union Pediatricians,* MEDGIS, 1948.

26. Pevzner, M.I., *Foundations of Therapeutic Nutrition,* MEDGIS, Moscow, 1949.

27. Pavlenko, S.M., *Some Questions in the Hereditary Pathology,* Contemporary Medicine, No. 2, 1955.

28. Pavlov, I.P., *Selected Works,* Moscow, Foreign Languages Publishing House, 1955.

29. Pershin, G.N., Makeeva, O.O., *Chemicotherapeutic Activity of Fthivasid,* Problems of Tuberculosis, No. 2, 1953.